This book is dedicated to all, especially ladies, who neglect their health and choose to suffer in silence

# GRANDPA'S TIPS ON STAYING HEALTHY WITH HOMEOPATHY, ALLOPATHY, TRADITIONAL MEDICINES AND SELF MEDICATION

COL (RETD) BHASKAR SARKAR

# Contents

*Preface* *vii*

1. Staying Healthy 1
2. Origin And Development Of Homeopathy 10
3. Homeopathic Medicines 18
4. Selection Of Medicines 24
5. Myths And Realities 27
6. Prevention Of Diseases 30
7. First Aid 43
8. Problems Of Mind, Head And Fevers 53
9. Problems Of Eyes, Ears, Nose, Mouth, Teeth And Throat 62
10. Problems Of Heart And Lungs 71
11. Problems Of The Digestive System 76
12. Problems Of The Urinary System 80
13. Problems Related To Rectum And Stool 83
14. Problems Related To Back And Locomotor System 86
15. Problems Of Skin 95
16. Women's Medical Problems 102
17. Sexual Problems Of Men And Women 112
18. Life Style Diseases 117
19. Problems Of The Aged 124
20. Problem Of Children 134
21. Arthritis, Gout And Rehumatism 140
22. Treatment Of Cancers 145

Epilogue 151

# Preface

**Staying healthy is our fundamental obligation to ourselves, our families and to society.** Just as there are many roads to Rome, there are many ways of staying healthy. It calls for a fair degree of self-control. The urge or motivation has to come from within. No one can force anyone to follow healthy life styles and habits. **This book explains Grandpa's method of staying fit. It is not the only way. Grandpa requests you to strive to stay healthy adopting your own way.**

Grandpa relies a lot on Homeopathy to stay healthy. **Grandpa decided to take up Homeopathy in 1988.** The provocation was Grandma falling ill on a Saturday night. The problem was not serious enough to merit getting her admitted to a hospital. Army doctors do not see out door patients on Sundays. So, she had to be content with taking off the counter pills till they could see the doctor on Monday and start on a course of treatment.

**Grandpa had also seen Homeopathy give some remarkable results.** In the early years after marriage, Grandma used to get annual attacks of "Pharyngitis" (a throat infection that came with a painful throat and fever and required a five-day course of antibiotics to cure the problem). One such attack took place when Grandpa was on annual leave at a small town in Assam to which Grandma belonged. They went to a Homeopath. He gave ten small white pills which were to be dissolved in a glass of water. She was to take one spoon of the liquid before going to bed, put one spoon of the liquid in a fresh glass and fill it with fresh water, and throw away the rest of the liquid. The process was to be repeated on the next two days. At the end of three days, Grandma was completely cured. That was in 1970. She has never had an attack of "Pharyngitis" again till date. Grandpa cannot prove that it was the result of efficacy of Homeopathic treatment or a matter of chance.

Army officers of College of Military Engineering, Pune, used to take their children to a Homeopath for their minor ailments. Some of Grandpa's army friends also prescribed Homeopathic medicines for free. So, **one fine day, Grandpa decided to study the subject and start using the medicines. He bought five books and about twenty commonly used medicines and launched into Homeopathy. Grandpa has never regretted the day.**

**Grandpa does not claim to be a great Homeopath.** But in the 34 years since 1988, he has treated many cases successfully. **On many occasions, Homeopathy has been in the nature of a temporary measure or first aid till**

**the patient could reach a doctor.** For example, once during a thunder storm close to midnight, a door slammed on the finger of a six-year-old boy. He started howling with pain. Grandpa put ice on the finger, gave him a dose of Arnica 1000 and Hypericum 30 and rushed him to the Military Hospital. It took them about thirty minutes to get there. By the time they reached, the medicine had taken effect and the boy had stopped crying.

**Many of us, poor or well to do, have spent hours or days or even months in remote areas where medical aid is not immediately available.** There are engineers and workers at construction sites in remote areas building dams, roads or hydroelectric projects. There are NGOs doing social work in remote villages. There are detachments of security forces deployed in inhospitable mountains or jungles. There are tourists trekking in the hills or visiting wild life sanctuaries. There are ordinary villagers, students, or professionals living, holidaying or working in remote areas where medical aid is not readily available. **Last but not the least, hundreds of thousand people under COVID-19 related lockdowns had no access to doctors or to any treatment. Homeopathy, over the counter drugs and self-medication are the only viable options in such situations.**

**Allopathic drug manufacturing companies sell trillions of dollars' worth of drugs at phenomenal profits. They run a slanderous campaign against Homeopathy and other traditional medicines.** If they had their way, they would also ban generic drugs because they are cheap and their availability reduces the sale of expensive drugs. **Fortunately, the Government of India and some other countries support alternate medicines and funds research in these professions.** India has established hospitals and colleges for training in alternate medicines like Homeopathy, Ayurveda (Indian traditional medicine) and Unani (Muslim traditional medicine). Many hospitals in India have departments offering treatment with Homeopathy and other alternate forms of medicine.

**This book is not a text book of Homeopathy. It is a manual for prevention, first aid and self-medication till a serious patient can access expert medical treatment.** It is a manual for self-medication for minor or unusual problems which do not always respond to allopathic treatment. It is also a manual for self-medication for those who cannot afford allopathic treatment or where the doctor says that the patient is incurable.

***All persons purchasing and using this book must realize that self-medication and Homeopathy have limitations which are explained in detail in Chapter 2. For all life-threatening diseases or injuries, the patient must***

***be evacuated to a hospital at the earliest possible. The first aid or treatment suggested is only a stop gap measure till expert medical facilities can be accessed. The author or the publisher does not accept any liability for self-medication or treatment suggested in the Book.***

**This is the Authors fifth book in the "Grandpa" series. The others, "Grandpa's Tips on Manoeuvring Through Life; Grandpa's Tips on Management for All; Grandpa's Tales: Ambush and Other Stories and Grandpa's Selection: Outstanding Victories of the Indian Army are available at Amazon, Flipkart or Notion Press.com.**

**Author**

**colbhaskarvsm@gmail.com**

**Contents**

Chapter 1: Staying Healthy
Chapter 2: Origin and Development of Homeopathy
Chapter 3: Homeopathic Medicines
Chapter 4: Selection and Incompatibility of Medicines
Chapter 5: Myths and Realities
Chapter 6: Prevention of Diseases
Chapter 7: First Aid
Chapter 8: Problems of the Mind and Head
Chapter 9: Problems of Eyes, Ears, Nose, Mouth, Teeth and Throat
Chapter 10: Problems of Heart and Circulatory System
Chapter 11: Problems of the Digestive System
Chapter 12: Problems of the Urinary System
Chapter 13: Problems Related to Rectum and Stool
Chapter 14: Problems Related to Back and Locomotory Systems
Chapter 15: Problems of Skin
Chapter 16: Problems of Women
Chapter 17: Life Style Diseases
Chapter 18: Problems of the Aged
Chapter 19: Problems of Children
Chapter 20: Arthritis and Joint Pains
Chapter 21: Cancers
Epilogue
Index of Diseases
Bibliography

# 1

# Staying Healthy

**Staying healthy is a challenge faced by most of us.** The environment we live in is totally against staying healthy. The air quality in most cities is poor. Quality of water is poor in many places. The use of RO removes many essential minerals from drinking water. Many of the food stuff including milk, cottage cheese and spices we buy are adulterated, often with cancerous chemicals. Hormones are injected into animals and vegetables to make them grow larger and faster to enhance profits. Cancerous pesticides are sprayed on most vegetables and fruits to keep pests away. Apples and some other fruits are coated with wax so that they stay fresh longer. Acids are used to clean root vegetables like potatoes and ginger. Formaldehyde is used to preserve meats and fish. Then there is the temptation of delicious fast foods which are usually bad for health.

**Stress, the prime killer**, is our constant companion. Competition starts in the kindergarten and continues to the grave. We are always trying to meet the expectations of others; children are trying to meet expectations of parents; workers expectations of bosses; husband and boyfriends of expectations of wives and girlfriends and vice versa. The ambitious amongst us are working day and night to achieve lofty goals. Then there are problems with lifestyle. Long working or study hours leave little time to spend with family or to exercise. Many of us spend long hours on the computer and mobile phone which is bad for the eyes and back. Stress often leads to drinking and eating disorders which are bad for health. Men, as young as 30 are dying from heart attacks.

**Grandpa has listed above some of the problems which we face in trying to stay healthy. But he is not trying to tell you what to do. He is not a doctor, dietician or psychologist. Who is he to tell you what to do?Grandpa's USP**

**is that he is a reasonably healthy 81 years old.** His hair is intact, he has not had a cataract operation or any prostrate problem. His teeth are gone and he had a stent placed in his heart in 2007. Both were possibly due to smoking which he started in 1962 and stopped in 2007. In this chapter, he is sharing his research and personal experiences in trying to remain healthy. He starts with tips on **eating healthy**.

**Our body needs a number of Vitamins and minerals.**

- Vitamin A (Retinol) is available in cheese, oily fish, milk products, liver (max 75g /week), eggs, oily fish (sardines, mackerel), fortified low fat spread, carrots, sweet potatoes, broccoli, orange or yellow fruits and vegetables which contain beta carotene like carrots. Men need .7mg/day; Women .6 mg/day. Max intake should not exceed 1.5 mg.
- Vitamin B 1(Thiamine). It is available in ham, soya milk, water melon etc. Men need 1 mg/day; women .8mg
- Vitamin B 2 (Riboflavin). It is available in milk, yogurt and cheese. Men need 1.3 mg/day; women 1.1 mg. Max intake should not exceed 40 mg.
- Vitamin B3 (Niacin). It is available in meat, poultry, fish, mushrooms and potatoes. Men need 16.5 mg/day; women 13.2. Max intake should not exceed 500 mg.
- Vitamin B6 (Pyridoxine). It is available in meat, fish, poultry, pulses, soya products & bananas. Men need 1.4 mg/day; women 1.2 mg. Max intake should not exceed 10 mg.
- Vitamin B7 (Biotin). It is available in eggs, soya products and fish. Daily intake should not exceed 0.9 mg.
- Vitamin B 12. Available in meat, fish and poultry. Daily intake recommended is 1.5 mcg; max 2 mg.
- Vitamin C. Available in citrus fruits and green vegetables. Recommended daily intake is 500 mg; max 1000 mg.
- Vitamin D. Sunlight exposure most important, milk products, cereals & fatty fish. Recommended daily dose is 40 mcg; max 100 mcg.
- Vitamin E is available in vegetable oils and nuts. Recommended daily intake for men is 4 mg and women 3 mg. Max 540 mg.
- Vitamin K is available in Cabbage, eggs, milk, spinach, broccoli, cucumber, and cauliflower. Recommended dose is 1 mcg/kg of weight; max 1 mg.
- Boron is available in Chickpeas, almonds, beans, bananas, walnuts, avocado, broccoli, apples & raisins.

- Calcium is available in yogurt, cheese and leafy vegetables.
- Chloride is available in salt.
- Magnesium is available in Spinach, pumpkin seeds, curd, almonds & dark chocolate
- Potassium is available in meat, shrimp, milk, fruit and pulses.
- Sodium is available in salt and soya sauce.
- Chromium is available in meat, poultry, fish, nuts and cheese.
- Copper is available in prawns, nuts and beans.
- Fluoride is available in fish and tea.
- Iodine is available in iodized salt and sea food.
- Iron is available in red meat, eggs, apples, banana, green vegetables, boiled raw banana
- Magnesium is available in nuts, dates and tea.
- Selenium is available in organ meats, sea food and walnuts.
- Zinc is available in Spinach, pumpkin seeds, curd, almonds, prawns & dark chocolate.

**Vitamins A, D, E and K are fat soluble.** Some fat in the form of butter or vegetable oils is essential for the body to absorb these vitamins. Hence, we have the Western custom of using salad oil and the Indian custom of taking mustard oil with boiled vegetables, eggs and pulses. Some form of fat has been used in recipes since ancient times.

It is important to know the symptoms and reasons for **vitamin D deficiency**. The main symptoms are whole body/muscle pains and feeling tired most of the time; frequent infections due to weakened immune system. **The primary reason for Vitamin D deficiency is inadequate exposure of the body to the sun**. Avoid going into the sun from 10 AM to 4 PM. UV rays are highest during this time. If you are able to expose part of your body to the sun for 30 minutes a day before 10 AM or after 4 PM, you will not have vitamin D deficiency. Diet alone cannot meet your need for Vitamin D. Sun exposure or Vitamin-D supplements are necessary. Food rich in phytates like whole grains, nuts, seeds and legumes and oxalates which are plenty in dark green leafy vegetables deplete Vitamin D in the body. Eating too much leafy vegetables and whole grains is not good for those who have Vitamin D deficiency, particularly ladies. Vitamin D needs some other vitamins and minerals to work. These are Magnesium, Vitamin K, Zinc, Boron and Vitamin A. If you are deficient in Vitamin D, you should ensure you take enough of the above vitamins in your food or as supplements.

Vitamin D is also essential for absorption of calcium by the body. Vitamin D Levels are very important for all Diabetics. Vitamin D deficiency leads to decrease of insulin secretion by up to 48%. Vitamin D directly acts on insulin producing cells in the pancreas to produce more insulin. Vitamin D reduces inflammation which is commonly present in patients with Insulin Resistance Syndrome and Type 2 diabetes.

Let us now know about **vitamins and minerals which are good for the eyes.** Ten foods which are a must for healthy eyes are fish (particularly **those rich in Omega 3 acids** like sardines, mackerel and other oily fish), nuts rich in Omega 3 Acids like walnut, cashew nuts, pea nuts, pulses, seeds (chia, flax, hemp), citrus fruit, leafy greens (spinach, methi etc), carrots, sweet potatoes and eggs (**Lutein and Zeaxanthin**). One needs to include more **glutathione** and antioxidant-rich foods in one's daily diet. Glutathione rich fruits are grapefruit, strawberries, and avocados. Also, eat food rich in Lutein and Zeaxanthin like corn, greens, eggs, and turnip greens. These may help prevent both macular degeneration and cataract.

**Symptoms of retinal problems** are a sudden increase of **"Floaters"**. Floaters are the unusual spots in your vision. They may appear like black or grey particles scattered all over the place, or like strings and cobwebs intertwined. When the number of floaters seems to grow suddenly or exponentially, you should grow concerned. Other symptoms are:

- Sudden and annoying flashes of light that tend to make you feel uncomfortable.
- Tunnel vision is another symptom. Peripheral vision is either blurred or hazed. At times, it could be due to Glaucoma. However, it is also one of the signs of retinal detachment.
- Deteriorating vision or seeing a swaying black or grey curtain. Distorted images are clearly manifestations of a possible damaged retina. Injury in the eye may also cause retinal detachment.

**Diet for persons suffering from cataract** should include a daily intake of Vitamin A 5,000 I. U., N-acetyl-cysteine 250 mg, Vitamin C 1000 mg, Vitamin E 800 I.U., Beta Carotene 25,000 I.U. Chromium 200 mcg. Zinc 15 mg. Rutina 250 mg. Quercetin Bioflavonoid 300 mg. Vitamin B-2 (Riboflavin HCL) 50 mg. Each person should formulate a diet out of the options available and take vitamin tablets or dietary supplements to get most of the needs.

**Vitamin A** is a powerful antioxidant known to help maintain healthy vision and skin. It is responsible for producing the pigmented layer of the retina that aids the light-sensing rods and cones of the latter to carry on with their functions.

**Carotenoids** are nutrients that make fruits and vegetables appear red, yellow, and orange. Carotenoids are found in the retina. Studies have shown that eating food with these nutrients lessen the chances of age-related macular degeneration (AMD) and cataracts. Food rich in carotenoids include eggs, broccoli, spinach, tomatoes, and zucchini. Omega-3 Fatty Acids are essential fats found in the eyes and brain.

**N-acetyl-cysteine**, a stable amino acid, has been shown to raise the levels of Glutathione. Cysteine is found in protein rich eggs. **Completely avoiding eggs may rob the body of this amino acid** which may have anti cataract properties. Eggs can increase cholesterol. However, cholesterol levels can be controlled by medicine. No other food is as effective in keeping our eyes healthy. Persons in teens should take two eggs a day. Old people must take an egg a day.

The lens of the human eye is bathed in a **vitamin C** rich aqueous solution which is 30 times more concentrated than the human blood. It appears that this vitamin C acts as an ultraviolet filter preventing the harmful effects of ultraviolet light. With age the levels of vitamin C begin to decrease and this may contribute to the formation of the senile cataract. There are several studies which have shown that high doses of vitamin C (1000 mg/ day) will reverse the development of some cataracts. High levels of Glutathione keep the human lens clear and prevent the development of cataracts. In one study, 81 percent of patients with cataracts were deficient in riboflavin.

Foods that produce **uric acid** should be avoided by those who suffer from **Arthritis and Gout**. These include red meat, organ meat, fatty poultry, bacon, fruit juices, aerated soft drinks and alcohol. Vitamin C reduces levels of uric acid. Do not give up on lean meats, fish, sea foods and alcohol. Reduce the quantity and frequency of these foods.

**Some form of exercise is a must.** Walking for half an hour a day five to six days a week is recommended by most doctors. "Pranayam" (a form of Yoga) is a very desirable form of Yogic breathing exercise which is very beneficial. Grandpa has practised it since 2007 when he had a stent inserted in his heart. But one should not overdo exercise. Grandpa recommends that the aged should enjoy exercising and not do what is tiring.

**Management of Stress** is essential for staying healthy. Stress can be avoided by controlling expectations, temper and ambitions, developing an attitude of gratitude and remembering "we win some and lose some." One should take failures and setbacks in their stride. **One should never brood over the past because the past can never be changed.** All we can do is learn lessons from the past. It is also ensured by living the life of a law-abiding citizen, avoiding greed and jealousy. Stress can be reduced by physical exercise, praying, listening to music, being with friends and family and doing things we enjoy. **Any attempt to reduce stress by snacking all day, smoking, chewing tobacco, taking drugs or excessive drinking will be disastrous. Having a healthy mental attitude like; "we win some and lose some"; "change is inevitable", "giving without expectations" and accepting what happens as the "will of God" will help manage stress.**

**Good and adequate sleep is essential for good health.** Seven to eight hours of sleep is required to stay healthy. However, many working in the corporate world, particularly in the IT sector find it impossible to get adequate sleep. Those working night shifts must get used to sleeping by day. Students must avoid studying late into the night or very early in the morning. The aged often tend to wake up very early in the morning. They must make up by sleeping in the afternoon or mid-morning to stay healthy. Watching TV late into the night is a bad habit and will have an effect on one's health. **Inadequate sleep can result in temporary loss of memory and weakness. It can also result in increased stress, migraine and even heart problems. Extreme sleep deprivation is form of torture used for interrogation of prisoners and terrorists.**

One should try to **prevent cancerous (cancer causing) substances from entering our body**. Avoid smoking, chewing tobacco, water stored in black PVC water tanks or old disposable plastic bottles. Grandpa recommends peeling all fruits and vegetables which can be peeled including soaking and peeling almonds to avoid insecticides and pesticides. He tries to buy freshly slaughtered meat and poultry and wash fish and greens very well in running water.

**Early detection of medical problems is essential for certainty of cure.** You are the only one who will know if you have a problem. Grandpa says, "Do not neglect minor problems or they will become major." Grandpa tests blood pressure once a month. He is non diabetic. He does lipid profile; liver function and serum creatinine (for kidney function) test every four months. Grandma is diabetic. She does "fasting" and PP sugar test once a month,

HBA1C once every 3 months and lipid profile, liver function and serum creatinine tests every 4 months. You can consult your doctor about tests and their frequency.

Grandpa would like to share with you hisway of staying healthy. He feels that it is difficult to calculate whether his diet has given him the vitamins and minerals he needs. So, he uses Becosules Performance multivitamin tablets. Grandma takes Nurokind Plus as advised by her doctor. They both take Lycored capsules, a dietary supplement containing Lycopene, zinc and selenium which is supposed to be a good antioxidant and beneficial for prostrate daily. There are many options available to select from. Grandpa takes a number of meals as given below:

7 AM Tea and Biscuits

9 AM Breakfast: 5 almonds soaked overnight with peel removed, fruit, porridge/corn flakes/dalia (crushed wheat) with milk, two toasts with one egg/one slice cheese/tinned sardines/mackerel and butter/ margarine and a glass of milk.

11 AM Some fruit and juice.

1 PM Lunch: Rice, dal or one vegetable, fish or egg dish and curd or raita

4 PM Tea and Biscuits

7 PM Whiskey and snacks

9 PM Dinner: 2 to 3 chapatis, dal or a vegetable dish and a paneer, chicken or egg dish

Grandpa tries to avoid stress by accepting events as the will of God. He **never looks at the past with regret but to learn from mistakes and never looks at the future with fear but to plan for it. He does not compare himself with others.** Grandpa and Grandma have learnt to appreciate others. Grandpa prays once or twice every day. But he does not go to religious places or sermons.

For exercise, Grandpa does "Pranayam" almost every morning and goes up and down 150 to 200 steps every day. He goes for walks when in the mood. He gets half an hour's exposure to sun while gardening. Grandma has recently been asked to do an exercise routine by a physiotherapist. She follows it religiously.

**There are different types of treatment for medical problems.** Baba Ramdev, yoga teacher; industrialist; political personality, has set a cat among the pigeons with his tirade against Allopathy. What is the truth?

Allopathy, Homeopathy, Ayurveda and other forms of traditional medicine like Unani (Muslim), Acupuncture (Chinese) etc. are in use and are relieving the suffering of millions of people every day. Allopathy is only about 300 years old. Human civilization is over 5000 years old. **The human race has survived nearly 5000 years without allopathy. All forms of medicines have limitations and are not infallible.**

It is not out of place for **Grandpa** to share his personal experiences. He **is not dogmatic and uses all forms of medicines**. When he had bouts of breathlessness in 2007, he did not try Homeopathy. He went and got ECG done. ECG showed a heart problem. He went to a hospital and got a stent inserted. **Grandpa does not go to alternate medicine for life threatening diseases involving vital organs.**

**In 1985, Grandma had a severe tennis elbow** and could not even put on her clothes. Grandpa got her treated at the Command Hospital, Kolkata for a month. All kinds of physiotherapy were done. There was no improvement. Finally, on recommendation of a friend, **they went to a traditional bone setter (Old world Orthopaedic specialist).** He put some liquid on the elbow and tied a bandage. The process was repeated two more times with an interval of a week. After 3 weeks she was completely cured. In 1993, **Grandpa's daughter had a severe attack of Jaundice while at Chennai. She went to a reputed Unani Jaundice specialist and was completely cured in a week.** When Grandma was found COVID positive with moderate infection recently in Chennai, she went into isolation and was treated with Favi Flu and a few other medicines. Grandpa also went into isolation with her so that she was not in solitary confinement. He gave her some Homeopathy medicines and took the same along with paracetamol, vit C and Zinco vit. **Grandpa lived 20 days with her in the room without even a mask without getting infected.** None of them had any major symptoms. CRP and D-Dimer tests show both to be COVID free.

Grandpa treats headache with Disprin, cough with Kuka syrup (Ayurveda), stomach upset with Pudin Hara (Ayurveda), Grandma's knee joint pain with Doctor Ortho, a message oil (Ayurveda) and occasionally paracetamol. He treated a bereaved lady and her son with Arnica to help them get over their grief and take the husband's body for funeral. He also gave her homeopathic medicines to stop her hallucinations with great success.

**Grandpa is not asking anyone to change their philosophy.** He is only trying to explain his.

**Prevention is better than cure.** Grandpa tries to improve his immune system by eating a high protein healthy diet; doing "Pranayam" in the morning, eliminate stress with **"It is for you to strive, it is for God to decide whether you succeed" Gita approach**; exercise without stress and preventive use of Homeopathy and Ayurveda. Every form of medicine, Allopathy or Traditional, works well for some problems and has limitations. None are infallible. Otherwise, no one would die from illness.

**Early detection and treatment can make all the difference between life and death.** This requires clinical tests at prescribed intervals and listening to your body. **Do not allow problems to aggravate by delaying treatment.** We go to a mechanic if the car AC is not cooling properly or the water tap is dripping. Why do we not go to a doctor when we have pain or discomfort and ignore pain. **We check air pressure of the wheels of our transport but not our blood pressure, sugar levels, kidney and liver functioning.**

**The acumen and dedication of the doctor and not his qualification makes a lot of difference.** May God give you the wisdom to select the right one for your medical problem.

**Life is full of contradictions.** A cardiologist says do not take eggs. Eye specialist says to take an egg every day. Grandpa's friend had violent pain in his thigh. A scan showed an old injury. One specialist said to walk only with a walker. Another said exercise and strengthen your muscles. My friend exercises but avoids putting stress on the knees and hip. **The middle path is the best path.**

**Finally, it is your body and your life. You are the only one who knows what you feel. Do what you want but do not neglect medical problems. May God give you the wisdom to do the right thing.**

# 2

# Origin and Development of Homeopathy

**There are four main streams of medical treatment widely available in India. These are Allopathy, Homeopathy, Ayurveda or traditional Hindu medicines and Unani or traditional Muslim medicines.** In addition, there are naturopathy, faith healing and grandma's solutions. In Grandpa's experience of about 60 years of adult life, Grandpa has seen all the above systems work. **The problem is not with the method of treatment. It is with the knowledge, acumen and integrity of those who practice and prescribe the medicines.**

Allopathic system of medicine is the most commonly used in developed countries and urban areas of India. Its practitioners claim that it is the most scientifically proven system. It is also a trillion-dollar industry which commercially exploits the patient to the maximum. A common medicine for allergy, Avil is available for Rs 1 (2 cents). Its modern equivalent, Allerga, costs Rs 11 (20 cents). Grandpa's 97-year-old, father had an eye problem. The doctor prescribed an injection which cost over Rs 2000. My brother, who accompanied him, told the doctor that he could not afford it. The doctor prescribed another which cost about Rs 150 and cured the problem.

**Many do not believe in homeopathy.** The most violent opponents of Homeopathy include Grandpa's brother who is not a doctor and his niece who is a doctor in the US. **Everyone has the right to choose his line of treatment. Homeopathy has its own merits, which will be obvious to those who have open minds. The first requirement is to understand Homeopathy.**

**Origin**

The **Homeopathic** system of medicine is one of the finest systems of cure available to mankind. It was **developed in Germany by a German physician practicing Allopathic medicine, Dr Samuel Friedrich Hahnemann in late 18$^{th}$ Century.** Dr Hahnemann found Allopathic medicines objectionable because he felt that Allopathic treatment did not cure but simply relieved the symptom. For example, constipation is relieved but not cured by laxatives. Fever is not cured but relieved with paracetamol or aspirin.

Dr Hahnemann started his experiments in Homeopathy in 1790 with 'China', a traditional drug made from a Peruvian bark. He found that he could make himself sick by taking four drachms of the medicine twice a day. He noted the scores of symptoms of his sickness which affected his mind and parts of his body from head to toe. He found that the symptoms produced in him were exactly the same as the diseases for which the drug was being used by practitioners of traditional medicine. He thus formulated the law of "Similia Similibus Curenteur" or "like cures like". This is also the same as the ancient Indian thought that poison in mild doses neutralizes poison. The same principle is used in development of many Allopathic vaccines. Dr Hahnemann also found that drugs in their natural form aggravated symptoms of the sickness. For example, Arsenic administer to a person in its pure form would kill him. So, he decided to dilute the drug by a method called 'Potencization'. To prepare a medicine of one potency, one part of the drug is dissolved in 99 parts of a solvent which is inert or non-medicinal by rubbing and shaking for at least one hour. The most commonly used solvents are sugar of milk or rectified spirit. To produce potency two, one part of potency one medicine is added to 99 parts of a diluent and rubbed and shaken for at least one hour. By repeating the process, the frequently used potencies of 1, 2, 3, 6, 30, 200, 1000, 10000 are produced. Higher the potency, more powerful is the drug. **It is perhaps the first real life use of "Nano Technology".**

The process of experimenting with traditional medicines and noting down the symptoms produced is known as "proving". The records of the experiments led to the preparation of Homeopathic "Materia Medica" which gives the symptoms produced or cured by each Homeopathic drug. The experiments were carried out on Dr Hahnemann and his pupils and other healthy volunteers. By the time Dr Hahnemann died in 1843, he had personally proven and used about 100 Homeopathic medicines. **In 1819, some German drug manufacturers brought a case against him. The court ordered him to stop distributing Homeopathic medicines. He however**

**continued to treat the rich and the poor with the help of a royal decree and played a significant part in containing a cholera epidemic in Western Europe in 1831-32.** The process of proving new medicines continues even today and many medicines have been added to the list of Homeopathic formulations available in Dr Hahnemann's time.

Homeopathy spread to England and other parts of Europe during the lifetime of Dr Hahnemann. It also spread to the US. **Dr J T Kent, one of the most well-known authorities on Homeopathy, was an American and taught Materia Medica at Hahnemann Medical College in Chicago USA starting 1889. Dr W A Dewey, another American authority on Homeopathy and professor, University of Michigan Homeopathic College, wrote the book "Essentials of Homeopathic Therapeutics" in 1894. Dr William Boericke MD is another renowned US Homeopath He was a professor of Homeopathy at the University of California. His book, 'Pocket Manual of Homeopathic Materia Medica and Repertory," a very popular and informative book, was first published in the US in 1927.** The first Indian edition of the book was published in Kolkata in 1961. Switzerland is a major manufacturer and exporter of Homeopathic medicines. It is not clear as to when or how Homeopathy arrived in India. But this form of treatment is very popular and many firms in India produce Homeopathic medicines and cosmetic products.

**Fundamentals of Homeopathy**

Study and understanding of Homeopathy is usually done in three parts, the Organon of Medicine, the Materia Medica and Therapeutics.

**Organon of Medicine**

"Organon of Medicine" is a book written by Dr Hahnemann. In it he tried to explain the philosophy on which Homeopathic treatment is based. As per him, the mission of the physician is to restore the sick to health. The cure should be rapid, gentle and a permanent restoration of the health of the patient. The disease should be annihilated completely in the shortest possible time and in the most harmless way (without any side effects). The causes which give rise to an illness or perpetuate it have to be removed. **Some salient aspects of the Organon of Medicine are given in the succeeding paragraphs.**

**Diseases should not be identified by a few symptoms but by all symptoms from the mind and head to the toe.** Allopathy admits that genetics play a part in ailment. For example, children of diabetic or those suffering from heart ailments are more likely to suffer from these diseases.

But while treating them, all are treated with the same medicines. Hahnemann insisted that individual personality must be considered while treating a patient. Hence Allopathy has one generic remedy for one problem. But Homeopathy has many medicines for similar symptoms. For example, if muscle pain increases with exertion the medicine is Bryonia but if it reduces with exertion, the medicine is Rhus Tox. **Homeopaths therefore have to study not only the symptoms of the disease on all parts of the body and mind but also individual traits and what aggravates or ameliorates the symptoms.**

**Selection of the right medicine is the key to effective Homeopathic treatment.** Homeopathic medicines are not like broad spectrum antibiotics. Each medicine has very specific symptoms and is more effective in a particular type of person. For example, a patient with rheumatic pain who sweats profusely in the head needs Calcarea Carbonica while one who does not may need Ledum. **If the selection of medicine is correct, a recently developed disease will disappear in a few hours to a few days. Older and more complicated medical problems will take longer time.** If there is too much delay in improvement, the choice of medicine could be wrong. It is also possible that the patient is not adhering to instructions.

The medicine should be administered in very minute does. This is achieved by "potencization" or dilution of the mother tincture. More severe the symptoms, higher the potency or more minute the dose. Allopathic treatment is just the opposite where the more severe the symptoms, the higher the milligrams of medicine per dose.

**Materia Medica**

"Materia Medica" are books or parts of books which describes the symptoms which the medicine could be used for. The description starts with the mental state and nature of the patient. There after it describes the effect of the medicine on various parts of the body starting from head in descending order to the toe. **Self-help books on Homeopathy usually condense this description and make it easier for laymen to select medicines.**

**Therapeutics**

Therapeutics is the application of the knowledge of Materia Medica in selection of medicines and treating of diseases. It includes tips on selection of medicines, sequencing, combining and dosage of medicines. This is the most difficult part of Homeopathy.

**Forms of Medicines**

Homeopathy is a system of medicine that uses natural substances. Metals like gold, silver, and platinum, minerals like sulphur, arsenic, lead and substances available in the plant or animal kingdom have been transformed by "potencization" into different medicines. The medicines are available in Homeopathic dispensaries in the following forms.

***Single Medicines.*** These are unique medicines like say Arnica or Cannabis Indica. The medicines can be in the form of pills or liquid. It is also sometimes prescribed in the form of powder. Mother tincture is a liquid, zero potency of Homeopathic medicines which is used for external applications or internal administration. Homeopathic medicines commonly used for cuts and burns like Calendula and Cantharis are also available as ointments.

***Mixtures.*** Some Homeopaths give mixtures of different medicines is the form of powders. However, this form of medicine is not available in Homeopathic dispensaries.

***Readymade Combinations.*** These are ready made combinations of Homeopathic medicines which have been designed for different diseases. All major manufacturers of Homeopathic medicines, both Indian or foreign have these disease specific combinations. They are available at all Homeopathic dispensaries and are quite popular. They can be used by laymen with the help of catalogues. They can be quite effective. **Grandpa has used these combinations to treat migraine of his son and kidney problem in a few acquaintances.**

***Tonics.***Tonics are supposed to strengthen the human body or its parts. Homeopathic tonics are available for various problems like hair fall, heart, liver or menstrual problems. Grandma has used these tonics to check hair fall and to increase vitality.

**Types of Doctors**

There are three types of Homeopaths. These are:

***Doctors Having a Degree in Homeopathy.***This category has attended a degree course in a Homeopathy college. **They are sometimes secretive and do not name the medicine or mixture prescribed. Prescription may not be issued.** The medicines are issued in powder form in paper packets for a particular duration. Some of them also have a tendency to prolong the treatment. Some of these doctors discourage their patients from seeing an Allopathic doctor and prohibit them from taking Allopathic medicine while taking Homeopathic treatment. Such doctors can be dangerous and are responsible for bringing Homeopathy into disrepute. Grandpa's brother-in-law is over 65 years of age. His teeth were giving problems. He had been under Allopathic treatment for some other problems and was troubled by the side effects. So, he had switched to Homeopathic treatment. My brother-in-law had the misfortune of being recommended to one such doctor. The doctor kept giving him medicines but was unable to control the pain. After almost a year of suffering, he could bear it no longer. He went to a dentist who removed the troublesome teeth and fitted a denture. He is now perfectly all right. Some of these categories of Homeopaths are egoists and discourage medical investigation and Allopathic or surgical treatment. **They can delay life-saving treatment till it is too late and should be avoided.**

***Doctors Having a Degree in Allopathic Medicine.***There are many Homeopaths who started as allopathic doctors with recognized degrees in Allopathic medicine. Dr Hahnemann, the founder of Homeopathy was one of them. The motivation behind the conversion is obscure. One such Homeopath we often went to at Pune converted because he could not cure his wife's arthritis with Allopathic medicines. **They are more likely to name the medicines in their prescription. They are also more likely to realize the gravity of the illness, get pathological investigations done and recommend switch to Allopathic treatment when necessary.**

***Doctors Not Having Formal Degree.***The third category consists of free lancers like Grandpa. They have an analytical mind and have studied Homeopathy as a hobby. They may also have a software for prescribing Homeopathic medicine. Many of them charge no fees. They have limited experience in view of their limited exposure and clientele. This category is generally open minded and understand their limitation. However, they should only be consulted only for non-life-threatening diseases.

**It does not matter which type of doctor you go to. What is important is that he must be effective. He must be able to solve the medical problem or at least provide relief to pain within a couple of days. If he cannot, the doctor should be changed.**

**Types of Diseases**

Diseases are broadly classified into two categories as under in Homeopathy:

***Acute Diseases.***These are short duration medical problems which occur due to infections, exposure to extreme weather conditions like heat or cold or over indulgence in food and drinks. Some examples of acute diseases are colds, influenza, dysentery, malaria etc. Acute diseases usually respond well to potencies 30 and above and require a few days of treatment. Some can be cured with a single dose of medicine.

***Chronic Diseases.***These are serious medical problems which develop over a long period of time. Some examples are diabetes, high or low blood pressure, heart, liver or kidney problems, back ache etc. They may take a long time to cure and are usually treated with low or high potency medicines.

**When one has or suspects to have a serious medical problem, one must see a qualified and experienced doctor.** The doctor can be an allopath, a homeopath, an Ayurveda or Unani. Professional doctors see many patients a day and can best assess the seriousness of the situation. **An allopath is perhaps the best because he is likely to get some clinical investigations done before he finalizes his diagnosis.** Once a diagnosis has been done based on clinical investigation, one can select homeopathic medicines along with allopathic treatment to get a quicker or cheaper cure.

**Alternate forms of medicine are not always best suited for life threatening diseases, particularly where surgery may be necessary. Self-medication with Homeopathic medicines can and should only be an interim or emergency measure.**

**Dangers of Self Medication**

Homeopathic medicines do not have serious and violent side effects which some Allopathic medicines can produce. Injection of penicillin to a person allergic to it can result in death. Thalidomide, a drug given to expecting mothers in UK a few decades back, resulted in large number of deformed babies being born. Most Allopathic medicines have some side effects. For example, use of medication for thyroid over a long period can cause calcium deficiency. Homeopathic medicines do not have any side effects. **Excess intake of a medicine can cause aggravation of the symptoms. In such cases the medicine should be immediately discontinued and the case referred back to the doctor.** There are antidotes for such situations. So, there is no risk to life or limb due to self-medication with homeopathic medicines. The worst that can happen is that instead of relief there could be some aggravation.

**The main danger from self-medication with Homeopathic medicines is that it may lead to delay in seeing a doctor till it is too late. Grandpa's brother may have died because he tried self-medication with Homeopathy for COVID 19 and delayed going to a doctor. Self-medication in case of life-threatening diseases like heart problems, persistent and severe abdominal pains, appendicitis, asthma attacks, diabetes, head injuries,**

**internal injuries, dehydration should never be done except as an interim first aid measure. Every effort must be made to get the patient to a hospital or a qualified doctor as early as possible.**

**Conclusion**

Homeopathy is a well-established form of medical treatment. It was developed in Germany and most of the authorities of Homeopathic medicines are Americans. Homeopathy is taught in many American universities like Michigan, California, Chicago and Missouri to name a few. **It has been in use in the developed world for more than 200 years. It has survived that long because it is effective.** Sceptics who decry Homeopathy do so either because they are ignorant about the benefits of Homeopathy or because they are afraid that increase in the popularity of Homeopathy will hurt their commercial interests.

**Homeopathy, like any other form of medical treatment, is as good as the doctor treating the patient.** If the doctor is good, if he knows his limitations and if he is not egoistic or greedy, he can be expected to cure you or refer you to a specialist or super specialist. Grandpa has a neighbour who was suffering from total lack of appetite and inability to hold the food taken. He saw a reputed allopathic doctor of the town and was under his treatment for about three months. But his condition kept worsening and he was reduced to a skeleton. Finally, against the wishes of his doctor, he went and got admitted at a reputed hospital in Mumbai. Scans revealed that he had some problem with his intestine. The affected section of the intestine was removed through surgery and he is absolutely normal. **Egoistic, greedy, inadequately qualified or careless doctors, no matter which stream of medicine they practice, can kill and get away with it.** Just because some patients under Homeopathic treatment have died does not mean Homeopathy is ineffective. **Patients under Allopathic treatment are dying in thousands every day.** Homeopathy is perfectly safe and effective. It is as effective as any other form of medicine. The Government of India runs advertisement to the effect on Government controlled Television channels and encourages people to get themselves treated through Homeopathy.

**Homeopathic self-medication or treatment is reasonably safe and simple.** It is cheap and free from side effects. It is an ideal interim solution till you reach a doctor as first aid or a life-saving solution if you cannot afford expensive medical treatment. All those who live or work in areas where medical aid is not easily available would be advised to buy this book, study this book carefully and keep a Medicine kit suggested in Chapter 3.

# 3

# Homeopathic Medicines

Homeopathic medicines are mostly made from natural substances and chemicals. They could be metals, minerals and their compounds or products of herbs, fruits, flowers or from the animal kingdom. Most of these medicines were in use in traditional medicines used in different countries before the advent of Allopathy. **Homeopathic medicines should be kept in a box in a cool, dry and dust proof place. They should not be stored in places with strong odours like perfumes.** The cap of the medicine phials should be kept tightly closed. The medicines can be in liquid or pill form. The liquid medicines are dosed in drops. Pills are dosed in numbers, usually four. The standard pill size is 20. The shelf life of Homeopathic medicines is supposed to be infinite. However, if there is any discoloration, the medicine should be thrown away. If medicines are easily available, they should be purchased one or two drams at a time and replenished when almost finished. When administering medicines in the form of pills, these should be placed on the tongue of the patient with the help of a stainless steel or plastic spoon or the cap of the phial. They should not be dispensed with fingers or from the palm to avoid contamination. **Another very effective way of dispensing medicine is to take 10 pills and dissolve them is half a cup of lukewarm water. The solution should be stirred with a stainless-steel spoon for 3 minutes and sipped over a period of 30 minutes.** The liquid should be kept in the mouth for 1 minute for maximum effect. If the medicine is in liquid form, six drops or as advised by the doctor should be poured into half a cup of lukewarm water and sipped as explained earlier. A properly chosen medicine should take effect in a few hours. If there is no effect within a day, the potency or dosage should be increased. If there is no improvement in the next 24 hours, the medicine prescribed should be reviewed and changed.

**Homeopathic medicines should be taken on an empty stomach or at least 30 minutes before or after meals.**

**Concept of Potencies**

As we have seen in Chapter 1, Homeopathic medicines are available in different potencies. Dr Hahnemann believed that medicines are more effective when used in minute quantities. So, he developed a process to dilute or as he called it "dynamize" the drug by a method called 'Potentization'. To prepare a medicine of potency 1, one part of the drug in traditional form (mother tincture) is dissolved in 99 parts of a solvent which is inert or non-medicinal by rubbing and shaking for at least one hour. The most commonly used solvents are sugar of milk or rectified spirit. To produce potency two, one part of potency one medicine is added to 99 parts of a diluent and rubbed and shaken for at least one hour. By repeating the process, the frequently used potencies of 1, 2, 3, 6, 30, 200, 1000, 10000 are produced. Higher the potency, more powerful is the drug.

**Use of Potencies**

**There are differing views on the use of potencies.** Some homeopaths rarely use medicines above potency 30. However, Grandpa is a follower of the school which feels that relief obtained is inadequate if the potency selected is low. For example, acute bronchitis may not respond to Bryonia 30 but Bryonia 200 is much more effective. Grandpa therefore do not use potencies below 30. For fear of Homeopathic aggravation, he does not use potencies over 1000 or 1M. If one is confident of his selection and the patient does not show improvement, one should change to a higher potency. Further, if improvement stops after a few days of medication, it is appropriate to increase the potency of the medicine to the next level, 30 to 200 or 200 to 1000. For children, ordinarily potency 30 is used. However, there is no harm in raising the potency if required. Potency 1000 should not normally be used more than once a day. They should be used at shorter intervals if cure is not achieved in one or two days.

**Sequence of Medicines**

Some traditional Homeopaths or Homeopaths of the old school believe in using a single remedy or medicine for an ailment and changing of medicine only after giving it adequate time to cure. This process takes time and the patient remains sick for a longer period of time if the selection of medicine or potency was not perfect. For example, some doctors will first prescribe Hepar Sulph for an abscess and if it does not give relief give Silesia. So, the cure takes longer than if Silesia was used at the beginning. Some modern

Homeopaths prescribe two to three medicines at the same time. This takes care of any error in selection of medicine and achieves quicker cure. Some times more than one medicine is used for treating some diseases. For example, Aconite and Ipecac are used alternately for treating an asthma attack. Influenzin and Gelesemium or Rhus Tox is used to treat Influenza. Arnica and Ruta are used together to cure sprains. However, while using more than one medicine at the same time, one has to ensure that the medicines selected are not incompatible or inimical to each other.

Dr Kent pioneered the use of multiple medicines in series for curing certain diseases. When multiple medicines are used, they should be used in a desired sequence. Some beneficial sequences while using a combination of common medicines is given below:

Sulphur 200 is often used to start treatment of persistent diseases. 10 pills are dissolved in half a cup of lukewarm water and sipped over 30 minutes. No other medicine is taken that day.

When treating flu, Influenzin is used first and is followed by the next medicine depending on the dominating symptoms.

Aconite should be used first when it is used with other medicines.

**Some sequences are harmful.** Some important examples are; Kreosotum does not follow Carbo Veg. Sulphur does not follow Lycopodium. However, Lycopodium follows Sulphur. It is also better to start with lower potencies and increase the potency as the cure progresses and not the other way.

**Dosage**

The question of dosage is a vexing problem. There are many schools of thought on the issue. **The most commonly used dose is four No 20 pills or six drops in one teaspoon of water in a cup, three to four times a day or as advised by the doctor.** One dose should be taken early morning on an empty stomach. If two or three medicines are taken, 30 minutes gap should be given between medicines. Grandpa is a forgetful person and always forgets to take medicines on time. He also likes his two pegs of whiskey in the evening and hence cannot take Homeopathic medicines in the evening. **Grandpa therefore recommends six pills twice a day so that the quantity of medicine taken per day remains more or less the same as in standard doses.**

**The second method is dissolving 10 pills in half a cup of lukewarm water and taking one spoon of the liquid every 15 minutes.** The interval can be increased as the condition of the patient improves. If two medicines are to be used alternately, they can be dissolved in separate cups and spoon full of medicine taken alternately.

**A third system of dosage is dissolving 10 pills in a glass of water.** Take one spoon of the liquid before going to bed, put one spoon of the liquid in a fresh glass and fill it with fresh water, and throw away the rest of the liquid. The process is to be repeated on the next two days. This system is uncommon but sometimes effective in permanently curing recurring medical problems like pharyngitis, tonsillitis, etc.

**Unless otherwise indicated, a dose in this book means taking 6 No.20 pills of the medicine.**

**Duration of Treatment**

In acute diseases, the treatment should continue till the symptoms disappear. In chronic diseases, the treatment is necessary for a longer duration which could extend from a month to six months in some cases.

**Ready Mixes and Tonics**

To make it easier for laymen and amateur Homeopaths to use Homeopathic medicines, almost all major producers of Homeopathic medicines have come up with a wide range of problem specific ready mixes and tonics. Companies like Bio-Force, Switzerland and Allen's Laboratories, Lords Laboratories, Bios Laboratories etc have these ready mixes and tonics which can be bought off the self from any Homeopathic dispensary. One can go to the shop and select what they need.

There is a very wide range of products in the market. Grandpa has used a few of them and found them useful. With so many products available in the market and selling, they must be effective. **The main advantage of these products is that you do not have to know much about Homeopathy to use them. The person at the Homeopathic dispensary will be able to advise you on the choice of brand and medicine for a particular ailment.** If they do not alleviate the problem within three to five days, go to a doctor.

**Incompatibility of Medicines**

**While using multiple medicines, care should be taken to ensure that the medicines selected are not incompatible or inimical to each other.** The complete list is available in "Pocket Book of Homeopathic Materia Medica" by William Boericke MD. Some extracts are; Acid Nitric is inimical to Lachesis; Apis is inimical to Rhus Tox; Asterius Rubens is inimical to Coffea Cruda; Belladona is inimical to Acetic Acid and Dulcamara, Calcarea Carb is inimical to Acetic Acid; Cantheris is inimical to Coffea Cruda, Carbo Veg is inimical to Kreosotum; Cocculus is inimical to Coffea Cruda; Ignatia is inimical to Coffea Cruda and Nux Vomica; Kali Bi is inimical to Calcarea

Carb; Lachesis is inimical to Acid Nitric and Dulcamara; Ledum is inimical to China; Lycopodium is inimical to sulphur, Merc Sol is inimical to Silesia; Phosphorus is inimical to Causticum and Sepia is inimical to Bryonia and Lachesis.

**Recommended Homeopathic Kit**

**Grandpa recommends two types of Homeopathic medicine kits namely family kits and organizational kits.** Family kit is smaller. It contains first aid medicines, commonly required medicines and medicines specific to medical problems of the members of the family or the area in which they are living. For example, families living in high altitude areas should stock medicines for medical problems of high altitude and extremely cold areas while organizations working in deserts should stock medicines related to heat stroke, snake and scorpion bite problems.

**Family Kit**

The medicines listed in the next paragraph are recommended to be part of the family medical kit. They should be in 2-dram phials. The lids of the medicines must be kept tightly closed. The medicines should be kept in a cool dry place away from areas like kitchen which produce strong odours.

The family kit should contain commonly needed medicines. It should contain 30 ml of mother tincture of Callendula for applying on cuts and abrasions; mother tincture of Cantharis for application on burns and scalds and Thuja for application on warts. It should also contain Size 20 pills of Aconite 30, Apis 1000, Arnica 200, Arnica 1000, Arsenic Alb 200, Antim Crud 200, Argentum Nit 200, Belladonna 200, Berberis Vulgaris 200, Borax 200, Bryonia 200, Cantharis 200, Carbo Veg 200, Cheledonium 200, Eupator Perf 200, Gelsemium 200, Glonoine 200, Hamamelis 200, Hepar Sulph 200, Hypericum 200, Influenzin 200, Ipecac 200, Kali Bi 200, Ledum 200, Lycopodium 200, Milifoleum 200, Merc Sol 200, Nux Vomica 200, Nat Mur 200, Pulsatilla 30, Rhus Tox 200, Ruta 200, Silesia 200, Sulphur 200, Veratrum Alb 200 and Veratrum Alb 1000.

If anyone in the family has dental problems, the family kit should have in addition Calcarea Flour 200, Kreosotum 30 and Hekla Lava 200.

If the family has senior citizens, the family kit should have Baryta Carb 200, Conium 200, Anacardium 200 and Abies Nigera 200.

If a family member has motion sickness Cocculus 200 should be added to the family kit.

If the family has a heart patient, the family kit should include Cactus, Crataegus, Digitalis and Camphor mother tinctures and Cactus 30,

Crataegus 30, Digitalis 30, and Arsenic Iod 30 in pills.

If the family has a member with a knee problem, the family kit should have Sticta 200.

If the family is in a snow bound area, the family kit should include Rhus Ven mother tincture and Agaricus 200.

If a family member suffers from hypertension, the family kit should have Veratrum Virde 200.

**Organizational Kits**

Organizations have to cater for a large cross section of people. They should hold almost all the medicines listed above and in 8-dram bottles.

**Diagnostic Kits**

Digital diagnostic kits are available these days for measuring blood pressure and sugar levels. Individuals who can afford these should acquire them. Organizations must hold these equipment's in their medical aid posts or first aid centres or offices.

**Conclusion**

The range of Homeopathic medicines is vast. The total list has more than 800 medicines. However, a kit of about 45 medicines is adequate for an amateur's first aid and medicine kit. The recommended medicines which should form the kit have been given above.

As stated at the beginning of this chapter, deciding on the dosage is a difficult thing. However, the readers of this book need not worry too much about it. The recommended doses will be specified when we talk of treatment of diseases.

**When using more than one medicine, care should be taken to ensure that the medicines are not incompatible and are taken in the correct sequence.**

# 4

# Selection of Medicines

**Homeopathic medicines are symptom specific and not disease specific.** For example, there are 25 Homeopathic medicines for headache. If the headache is frontal, comes early in the morning and is worse with motion, the medicine is Bryonia. If it is due to sun stroke or exposure to sun, the medicine is Glonoine. On the other hand, two tablets of aspirin will cure most headaches. **In Homeopathy, the same medicine is used for many diseases.** Most medicines affect our body from head to toe. For example: Arnica is used for mental shock, to reduce pain from injuries, angina pain etc. Glonoine is prescribed to cure double vision as also in flu or for body ache.

**Selection of medicine is the most difficult part of Homeopathy.** With about 75 to 100 commonly used medicines and thousands of symptoms, it is almost humanly impossible to remember which medicine should be selected. Grandpa does not trust his memory and mostly refer to books when dealing with a case.

**Use of Books**

Use of books for selection of medicine requires a good understanding of books on Homeopathy. The books can be classified into three main categories. These are Materia Medica, combination of Materia Medic and Repertory or Therapeutics and guide books. Books which are entirely Materia Medica like "Lectures on Homeopathic Materia Meica" by Dr. J T Kent or "Materia Medica" by Boericke are for those who are studying to be Homeopathic doctors. They are in great detail and contain detailed description of the effects of the medicine during proving. The Combination books are more suitable for beginners. In such books, the Materia Medica is condensed and it is easier to match the symptoms of the patient with those of the medicines. Guide books cover the diseases starting with those of the mind, head, eye, and down to the extremities, skin and fevers. They may contain abridged Materia Medica and Indices which help the layman or amateurs like me to find the disease and its cure. Most guide books will have four parts as given below. However, the sequence of the parts may be different.

- **Materia Medica.** A Materia Medica lists the medicines in alphabetical order. The symptoms noticed in the patient during proving are listed starting with the mind, then head, eyes, nose, ears, mouth, teeth, throat, heart or circulatory, lungs or respiratory, digestive systems, back and neck, urinary system, female, male, rectum, stool, extremities, skin, fevers, etc. At the end of the description of each medicine, modalities (what aggravates or worsens the symptoms and ameliorates or reduces the symptoms), relationship and recommended potencies may be indicated. Beginners should not spend much time on Materia Medica as it can be confusing. Study of Materia Medica is useful in finally selecting the medicine after we have narrowed down the choice of medicine to about three.
- **Therapeutic Index.** The therapeutic index lists ailments in the same order as the Materia Medica and lists the possible medicines along with the symptoms of the medicine. While selecting medicines, it is best to start with the therapeutic index. If the choice is obvious go for it. If the choice is not obvious, select two or three which seem most appropriate and further analyse them by referring to the Materia Medica and Modalities Index.
- **Modalities.** Modalities or what aggravates or worsens the symptoms and ameliorates or reduces the symptoms is an important indicator of the medicine to be selected. Let us take an example. The patient is suffering from aches and pains in the body. If the pain increases with exertion or any motion, in the morning, in warm weather and feels better by pressure or lying on the painful side or rest, the medicine is Bryonia. But if the pain gets better with exertion or motion, by warm application and change of position but gets worse during rest or sleep, in cold weather and with pressure, the medicine is Rhus Tox.
- **Generalities.** This is a separate index or chapter in some books. It is similar to the therapeutic index. It lists medical problems which can be common to different parts of the body or not specific to any part of

the body. Some examples are abscess, anaemia, cancer etc. It suggests medicines based on the cause of the problem or the part affected.

**Use of Internet**

These days one can get advice on selection of Homeopathic medicine on the internet. If you type "Homeopathic Treatment" on the Google Search Engine, it offers you a number of sites. If you type "Homeopathic medicines for diabetes" you will get about 72,500 hits. You can go through a few sites and find a medicine that matches the symptoms of the patient. In fact, you can get suggestions on medicines for every kind of medical problem including sexual problems.

**Guidance from Shops**

One can also get good advice from the proprietors of Homeopathic Medicine shops regarding medicines for diseases, particularly of the readymade combinations and tonics.

**Conclusions**

**Selection of the correct medicine and dosage is the most challenging part of Homeopathy.** However, this book does not seek to make you a Homeopathic doctor. **It seeks to help you to select the most appropriate medicine for your medical problem and also suggests the dosage.** So, relax and make use of suggestions in the succeeding chapters when the need arises. If you are unable to make up your mind as to which is the most appropriate, you can take two medicines with a gap of half an hour. You can take up to three different medicines simultaneously with half an hour gap between medicines. You have to make sure that the medicines are not incompatible. **If you do not get the desired relief in three days, try another medicine. If you still do not get relief, you need to see a doctor.**

The internet provides a wealth of information and guidance on the efficacy and use of Homeopathic medicines. Those who are familiar with the use of internet will find it easy to use it for suggestions regarding selection of medicines and deciding on the line of treatment. It also saves on the expense of purchasing too many books. However, possession of one good guidebook is desirable

# 5

# Myths and Realities

There are a number of myths related to Homeopathy. Some of the myths have been created by Homeopaths themselves to increase their importance, propagate their views against use of alcohol or serve their commercial interests. Opponents of Homeopathy have also added their myths. Here we will deal with some of them.

**"Homeopathy Takes a Long Time to Cure"**

**This myth has been propagated by both Homeopaths and their opponents.** Let me narrate an incident. A few years after I had started on Homeopathy, my friend and his wife came visiting and we started discussing my new found interest. My friend's wife said that she had a back problem for which she was taking medicines from a renowned Homeopath who used to visit our town once every month from Mumbai. She could not bend forward and doing household chores like sweeping or making the bed which involved bending forward was very painful. The doctor used to charge Rs 50 or $2 (Rs 50 in 1989 was much more than what it is today) and give medicines for one month. This had been going on for six months and the improvement was negligible. The doctor had said that the problem would take time to cure. I told her that as per my studies, Homeopathic treatment worked fast. I brought out my books and selected a medicine which she agreed to try. She felt much better within 24 hours and was completely cured in about a week.

**If the correct medicine in the required potency is taken, Homeopathy, particularly in the case of acute diseases, shows positive improvement within 24 hours and cures completely within a couple of days.** One dose of ten pills of Veratrum Alb 1000 is supposed to cure Cholera. I have never had a chance to treat cholera. But I have stopped rice diarrhoea with one dose of Veratrum Alb 1000.

**Grandpa has personally experienced the quick action of Homeopathic medicines.** Once while on a tour of cyclone affected Orissa in 2000, he suddenly had a severe attack of loose motion and vomiting around midnight. He was staying at a small hotel at a small town. He treated himself with Arsenic Alb and Merc Sol and was all right by 10 o'clock the next morning and fit enough to continue the journey. Grandpa has seen pain from bee sting subside in an hour after taking Apis Mel 1000, toothache subside within hours after taking Hekla Lava 200 and Merc Sol 200.

**Chronic diseases like diabetes, heart problems, kidney disorders etc can take a long time to cure.** But for most common problems, Homeopathy can cure within days if not in hours. If a Homeopathic doctor tells you that treatment will take a long time and does not tell you what medicine and potency he is giving, he is taking you for a ride.

**"Initial Aggravation is Normal in Homeopathic Treatment"**

**This myth has been spread by Homeopaths themselves as a face-saving measure when they fail to select the proper medicine or potency.** Once my son had an attack of scabies and we took him to a Homeopath. He gave some medicine and the rashes erupted all over the body and started oozing. We went back to the doctor. He said that it was normal and the boy will be all right. We waited another day and when there was no improvement, took him to the hospital and got him admitted.

Homeopathic aggravation does occasionally occur if the dose given is too high or a combination of two medicines inimical to each other has been used by mistake during treatment. But if the doctor says that the aggravation is normal and because the medicine is taking effect and does not change the medicine, he is lying.

**"Homeopathic and Allopathic Medicines cannot be Used Together"**

**This myth has also been spread by Homeopaths to prevent their clients from going to Allopathic doctors for treatment.** There is absolutely no truth in the myth. In fact, some Homeopathic books recommend that you take Arnica 1000 before surgical operation or tooth extraction. This reduces pain, prevents pus formation and hastens cure. I have consistently used both Homeopathic and Allopathic medicines at the same time. **Relief to the patient is what is important. It does not matter whether the relief comes from Homeopathic or Allopathic medicines.**

**"Drinking and Homeopathy Do Not Go Together"**

**Many Homeopaths prohibit taking alcohol when taking Homeopathic medicines.** Grandpa has found no evidence to support this myth. He takes two pegs of whiskey almost every evening. Homeopathy works wonders for him. Of course, the fundamental rule that Homeopathic medicines should not be taken within 30 minutes of taking food or drinks apply.

**"Homeopathy is not based on Scientific Experiments"**

**This myth is spread by Allopathic doctors and drug companies to further their commercial interests.** In fact, a junior doctor's association in UK called Homeopathy witchcraft and recommended that it should be banned. **Homeopathy is not a traditional system of medicine originating in the Third World. It originated in Germany and was refined in the United States.** Most authorities on Homeopathic treatment are Americans. Homeopathy is taught in many American Universities and practiced in the US. The Ministry of Health and Family Planning, Government of India recognizes it, recommends its use and funds Homeopathic hospitals and colleges. So, **if you do not want to use Homeopathy, you are welcome not to. But why discourage others**?

**Conclusion**

**Commercial interests of doctors, both Homeopathic and Allopathic influence their attitude towards Homeopathy.** The commercial interests of the drug companies, who control a multi-trillion-dollar market, are overwhelming. They can influence WHO to overstate the threat from H1N1 virus so that their sales improve. They can influence the Government of India to close down all Public Sector vaccine producing units instead of upgrading them. They bribe doctors with gifts and holidays to encourage them to prescribe expensive medicines instead of cheaper generic versions. It is only natural that they would try to discourage Homeopathy as a method of treating diseases because homeopathic medicines are cheap. Homeopathy offers a cheap and hassle-free cure for many minor and unusual medical problems.

# 6

# Prevention of Diseases

**Prevention of diseases is certainly better than cure.** A balanced diet, adequate exercise, proper stress management and avoiding bad habits like smoking, excessive drinking, addiction to drugs and chewing tobacco does help in increasing body resistance and prevention of diseases. But this is not always enough. To prevent attack by some infections and viruses, it is advisable to take suitable vaccines and administer them to our family members. Common Allopathic vaccines like DTP, polio drops must be administered to children as per the prescribed immunization program of the government. Tetanus injection must be administered after cuts and abrasions where there is a danger of tetanus infection. Anti-rabies injection must be taken if bitten by unknown animal like dogs, monkeys etc. **Homeopathy claims to have many medicines which are supposed to prevent diseases.** Grandpa uses the word **"claims"** because there is no way to prove that a person was not infected due to taking a Homeopathic medicine. However, **Grandpa believes that there is no harm in taking a few pills if it can prevent a disease or a tragedy.**

**Grandpa's Approach to Prevention of Diseases**

**Grandpa says that all infections and diseases have a gestation period before the symptoms start appearing.** During this period, the body's immune system fights the invading infection or virus. Flu takes a few days, cancer possibly many weeks. During this stage, the germs or viruses are less entrenched and easily tackled. **If we could guess what is wrong at this stage, we can try to destroy the infection. You cannot take a prescription drug unless the doctor declares you sick. But you can take a Homeopathic medicine.** For example, if you are going to the urinal more than once at night you may be having a prostrate problem. You can take six pills of

Conium 200 twice a day and nip the medical problem in the bud. Food supplements can also help the body's immune system to fight off the infection or virus.

**Banishing Fears**

The human mind has many kinds of fears. Homeopathy offers medicines for overcoming these fears. The various types of fears and their medicines are as under:

- **Fear of death.** Aconite 30 or 200 and Arsenic Alb 200 in extreme cases. One dose of 6 pills dissolved in half cup of lukewarm water before going to sleep.
- **Fear of examination.** Take 6 pills each of Anacardium 200 and Argentum Nitricum 200 two times a day for 3 days prior to the start of the examination.
- **Fear of failure and lack of self-confidence.** Argentum Nitricum 200. Take one dose of 6 pills two times a day for 3 days before an interview, journey or a sports event. My wife always feels very uneasy before a journey and a dose of Argentum Nitricum the evening before invariably soothes her nerves.
- **Fear of being left alone.** One dose of Phosphorus 200 and one dose of Arsenic Alb 200 four hours before being left alone.

**Getting Drunk**

Sometimes, we attend parties where there is a chance of getting drunk or having a hangover later. **To avoid getting drunk or having hangover, take one dose of Nux Vomica 200 about one hour before the party.** A well buttered toast topped with a fried egg a few minutes before leaving for the party also helps by delaying absorption of alcohol into the system and reduces the chances of getting drunk.

**Suicide**

Suicidal tendencies can occur due to extreme hopelessness and despair. Some common situations and suggested remedies are given below. **It is very important that the person is not left alone after the mental shock for 24 to 48 hrs. Depression in any person should not be taken lightly.** Every effort has to be made to get the person to open up about his or her problem and discuss it. Sometimes, just sharing one's sorrow or fearsreduces depression. Physical exercise, playing games or listening to music can help.

- **Hopelessness due to failure in examination or not getting a job.** One dose of 6 pills of Aur Met 200 two times a day for three days immediately after the bad news. **Every effort also needs to console the person instead of chiding the person. Ensure that the person is not left alone.**
- **Due to mental shock due to death of spouse or child, financial loss, discovering infidelity on part of spouse or break up of marriage.** Dissolve 10 pills of Arnica 200 in a cup of water and administer one spoonful every half hour till night fall. Make the medicine again if it finishes.
- **Due to prolonged illness.** Carbo Veg 200 one dose three times a day for a month.

**Colds**

Some people have a tendency to catch a cold. Some common causes and preventive medicines are given below:

- **Tendency to catch cold at every change of weather.** One dose of Sulphur 200 and Calcarea Carb 200 on empty stomach once a week on different days for one month in spring, summer, onset of monsoons and onset of winter.
- **Tendency to continuously suffer from attacks of cold.** One dose of Nitric Acid 200 once a week on empty stomach for three months.
- **Running Nose.** One dose of Arsenic Alb 200 for two days.
- **Sore Throat.** Take cough syrup, one tablet of Paracetamol 650 mg and a vitamin C tablet at the first hint. If patient has a history of Tonsil, give one dose Baryta Carb 200 for two to three days.

**Bad Breath**

Unpleasant odour emanating from the mouth can be prevented by the following medicines depending on the cause of the problem:

- **Due to unhealthy gums:** One dose of Merc Sol 200 two times a day for three to five days. Repeat if required.
- **Due to pyorrhoea:** Silicea 200 one dose three times a day for three to five days. Continue if required.

**Dementia and Alzheimer's Disease**

These are diseases of the aged and are discussed in detail in Chapter Problems of the Aged. It occurs after the age of 65. The first indication is loss of memory, inability to remember names and recent events like dates of future events, appointment, etc. The person should be put on a healthy high protein diet and increase in physical activities and social interaction. One dose of six pills of Homeopathic medicines Baryta Carb 200 and Anacardium 200 should be given twice a week till there is visible improvement.

**Diphtheria**

**Diphtheria is a serious highly infectious problem of the throat which can lead to heart failure and death.** It can be prevented by immunization. Children are supposed to be immunized in the first year. The main symptoms are sore swollen throat and difficulty in breathing. One must see a doctor at the earliest. Apis 30 is supposed to prevent Diphtheria. One dose of 10 pills should be given to all persons in the house if there is a case in the family or neighbourhood.

**Mumps**

**Mumps is caused by a viral infection which leads to salivary glands.** There is swelling in front of and below ears. There can be inflammation in breasts, ovaries or pancreas in women and testes in men. **It is highly infections.** The preventive is Trifol 30 and Pulsatilla 30. One dose of 10 pills of each should be taken once a week if cases are occurring in the neighbourhood. Every effort must be made to take the patient to a hospital at the earliest.

**Tetanus**

Tetanus is a serious life-threatening disease caused by bacterial infection which takes place through cuts, punctures or abrasion caused by falls on roads or cuts or punctures while working with rusted or dirty metals tins, knives, nails etc. The patient experiences stiffness, pain in jaw, high temperature, headache and sweating. Ledum 200 is the preventive. Take one dose of 6 pills as early as possible after the injury. Get tetanus injection if available.

**Tonsillitis**

Swollen tonsils are accompanied by high temperature, white coated tongue, dry cough and bad breath. The problem is common in children. **It can be prevented by one dose of Baryta Carb 1000 once a week for three months.**

**Heart and Circulatory Systems**

Heart problems affect most persons as they age. The risk increases in people with sedentary habits, who are obese, diabetic and who smoke. The main early indications of impending heart problem are high levels of cholesterol and triglycerides in blood, high or low blood pressure, weak or irregular pulse rate, dyspepsia or breathing difficulty for short periods, sudden blackouts and extreme breathlessness and exhaustion on least physical exertion. **Regular check-ups are advisable after the age of 30 for those who can afford it.** Heart problems can arise from infections, blocking of arteries, degeneration of heart muscles or from mal function of heart valves. **High blood pressure or hypertension is one of the main reasons of coronary heart diseases. 120/80 is normal. 150/90 is high. 170/95 is dangerously high. Low blood pressure, say less than 90/60 accompanied by a pulse rate below 45 could mean that the heart is weak and unable to pump the required quantity of blood.** Prevention of heart diseases involves controlling high blood pressure by use of medicines and **blood thinners; control of cholesterol by drugs and fibre in diet.** Homeopathy also has drugs which can control blood pressure and cholesterol. Patients with weak heart need to improve their strength and stamina. Ultimately, they may need a pace maker.

Heart problems in patients with high blood pressure can be prevented with Crataegus 30 and Veratrum Viride 30. Crataegus is said to have solvent power upon deposits in arteries. Veratrum Viride reduces both systolic and diastolic blood pressure. 6 pills of Crataegus 30 mixed in half a cup of water and 6 pills of Veratrum Virde 30 should be taken two times a day continuously to prevent an attack. Veratrum Virde can be stopped if the blood pressure falls below 140/90. One can also take a blood thinner like Ecospirin 150 mg or 75 mg.

Heart problems in patients with low blood pressure or weak heart muscles can be prevented with Crataegus mother tincture and Digitalis 30. 10 drops of Crataegus mixed in half a cup of water and 6 pills of Digitalis 30 should be taken two times a day continuously to prevent an attack.

**Cholera**

If one is in the midst of a cholera epidemic, one dose of 10 pills of Cuprum Met 30 and Veratrum Alb 200 should be taken alternatively once every week as long as the epidemic lasts. The dose of Cuprum Met 30 should be taken first. This should be followed by the dose of Veratrum Alb 30.

**Diarrhoea**

If there is a diarrhoea epidemic after floods or due to contamination of drinking water Sulphur 200 acts as a prophylactic. One dose of 10 pills should be taken once every week as long as the epidemic lasts.

**Prostrate Atrophy or Cancer**

The prostate gland is located just below the bladder in men. It produces seminal fluid and controls the passage of semen during intercourse. Prostrate problem affects many men over 50. The early symptom is urinating more than once at night. Neglected, it can lead to atrophy or even cancer. Lycopene, present in red fruits and vegetables like tomatoes, helps in keeping prostrate healthy. It is also available in some food supplements like Lyco Red. Grandpa believes taking one dose of Conium 200 every week prevents prostrate problems. Keeping the gland active by self-gratification could also prevent prostrate problems.

**Kidney Stones**

Kidney stones are a common problem in areas where water contains a lot of dissolved impurities. Grandpa believes that taking one dose of **Berberis Vulgaris 200** every week will prevent formation of kidney stones.

**Gall Blader Stones**

Stones in gall bladder is another common problem. These stones were detected in Grandpa in 1988 during sonography and he went to the Armed Forces Medical College, Pune, to get it removed. There he was told that there is no need to operate unless there is pain. Grandpa has been taking **Berberis Vulgaris 200 and Calcarea Carb 30** once a week to keep the stones away. Grandpa's gallbladder stones have not become painful as yet. He does not know if they are still there. The stones if small pass into the stomach and out with stool if butter and oil is a part of the diet.

**Liver Problems**

It is difficult to detect liver problems at an early stage. Periodic liver function test can be one option. **Berberis Vulgaris, Chelidonium and Phosphorous** give relief for most liver problems. These medicines could be taken once a week to prevent liver malfunction.

**Abortion or Miscarriage**

Miscarriage can be due to injury like a fall or an accident. One dose of Arnica 200 should be administered as early as possible after an injury to pregnant women to avoid abortion. Every attempt must be made to get to a doctor.

**Some women have a tendency to miscarriage.** Such women should be given one dose of Sabina 30 once a week from the third to the eighth month to prevent miscarriage.

**Diabetic Gangrene**

Gangrene is a disease where tissues of the body die after their food supply is cut off by bacterial infection. Injuries like cuts and pierced wounds and even internal injuries due to accidents do not heal easily in diabetic persons. **If neglected it may lead to gangrene which in turn may lead to amputation.** Gangrene in diabetic persons can be prevented by taking Arsenic Alb 200 along with other medicines. One dose of 6 pills should be taken two times a day till the wound heals. The dosage should start immediately after first aid has been administered. The subject will be elaborated when discussing diabetes.

**Septic**

One dose of Arnica 1000 should be taken before one goes for tooth extraction, operation and child birth to reduce pain and to prevent the wounds becoming septic.

**Sweating**

Some persons have a tendency to sweat profusely. Some medicines which reduce sweating are given below. One dose of 6 pills should be taken once a day during the sweating season.

- **Sweating in the head**, hair is wet: Calcarea Carb 30.
- Sweat is sour with offensive odor: Hepar Sulph 200
- Sweat is oily and sticky sweat: Merc Sol 200
- Only upper body sweats: Opium 200
- Sweating with burning in arm pits and leg pits: Sulphur 200

**Fevers**

**Hay- Fever**

Hay fever is an allergy caused due to pollens in the air. There is fever and running nose. One dose of 10 pills of Arsenic Alb 200 should be taken once a week in the hay fever season.

**Influenza or Flu**

Influenza results from a viral infection of the respiratory tract. The other symptoms can include general weakness, body pain, pain in bones, sneezing, coryza and fever. Recently there was a Flu epidemic caused by the H1N1 or Bird Flu virus. If not controlled, it can lead to pneumonia and death. **The preventive is Influenzin 200.** Six pills should be taken in the morning and another six in the evening on the same day when incidence of flu is reported in the locality, school, place of work or when traveling by public transport. **Some recommend taking one dose of 10 pills of Arsenic Alb 200 the next day.**

**COVID 19**

The Corona Virus is a virulent virus that spreads by personal contact or contact with the virus while it is alive on any surface like skin, railings, lift buttons, clothes, upholstery of public transport etc or through saliva thrown into the air while talking or sneezing. It usually first arrives on the hand and from the hand it passes into the mouth or nose and from there into the lungs or the urinary system. It is most lethal for the aged and those suffering from other serious s diseases like diabetics, heart problems etc. It kills by causing severe pneumonia, kidney or multi organ failure. The mortality rate is low. It is about 1% of those infected except for persons over 65 and those with existing serious medical conditions like diabetes, kidney or liver problems. The casualty rate is likely to reduce as doctors around the world gain more experience in dealing with it, more infrastructure like ventilators, oxygen and ICU beds become available and medical research finds vaccines and medicines for the disease.

**For COVID 19 to spread, three conditions must be fulfilled.** Firstly, there must be an infected person nearby to provide the infection. Secondly, there must be persons within two meters of the infected person to whom the infection can spread by direct contact of hands or by spray of saliva. Thirdly, a healthy person must touch a surface infected by an infected person. **It is best prevented by social distancing, isolation of infected persons, frequent sanitizing of hands and using protective gear like masks and gloves whenever going out.**

**We have to understand the implications of vaccination.** Vaccines increase immunity against a particular disease. They take many years to develop. The vaccines for COVID 19 which are in use today have been developed and brought into use in a hurry without adequate trials. **No one knows how effective they are. So, the medical authorities insist that those who have taken the vaccine must also take full protection. Grandpa's brother who had taken both doses of the vaccine died of COVID-19.** Grandma, who had her first dose, tested COVID positive with moderate infection and was cured during isolation. Grandpa had had the first dose. He spent the entire two weeks of isolation in the same room as Grandma to give her company and keep her morale high. He did not get affected. The reason could be that the vaccine did not work for Grandpa's brother or Grandma but it worked for him.

**When the makers of a vaccine say that a vaccine is 80% safe, it means that out of 100 vaccinated, 80 are safe and 20 are not. No individual knows whether he or she is safe or not.Hence all individuals must take all precautions.** Then why do governments spend so much money to get their population vaccinated. It is because with their population vaccinated the no of patients will be less. Less medical infrastructure will be required. The death figures will be lower and they will earn kudos from the electorate and the world. **Please cooperate with the government. Take your two jabs.** You may be lucky like Grandpa and be safe. Grandpa has taken his second jab. It will not be for protection but to be able to travel freely.

**Homeopathic medicine Camphora 1M has been recommended by renowned industrialist, Mr. Rajib Bajaj as a preventive.**He has given it to all his over 10,000 employees. Take 4 pills first thing in the morning on empty stomach for three days running and then one dose every 7 days for three weeks. If Camphora 1M is not available, you can use 6 pills of Camphora 200 pills as Grandpa has done. **Some recommend Arsenic Alb 200, the same way. One can even use both.**

**Intermittent Fevers**

Intermittent fevers include Malaria and Typhoid. The first is caused by infection through mosquito bite. The second is due to water borne infection. Both are common during rainy season. One must take precautions to prevent mosquito breeding and bite. One must boil water before drinking if water purifiers are not being used. **The preventive is Arsenic Alb 200. One dose of 10 pills should be taken once a week during rainy season.**

**Measles**

Measles is a highly contagious viral infection which occurs mostly in childhood. The symptoms are high fever, running nose and cough. Rashes appear all over the body after about four days. The preventive is one dose of 6 pills of Aconite 30 followed by one dose of 6 pills of Pulsatilla 30 if cases of measles are reported in the locality or school.

**Children**

**Whooping Cough**

Whooping cough is a severe cough which can affect infants and children not immunized against it. At the end of a spasm of severe coughing, there is a sharp, noisy intake of breadth. The preventive is Drosea 30. One dose of 4 pills should be given once a week to children who have not been immunized when a case occurs in the locality.

**Motion Sickness**

Some people get nausea with vomiting when traveling by road, rail, sea or air. **This can be prevented by taking one dose of 6 pills of Cocculus 200 one hour before the start of the journey.** If the journey is a long one, the dose can be repeated every four hours.

**Pus formation**

Simple wounds or cuts can get septic and there is pus formation. The situation becomes complicated and difficult to cure. This pus formation can be prevented by taking one dose of 4 pills of Arnica 1000 after the injury or before an operation or tooth extraction.

**Tetanus**

If a wound or abrasion is caused by an unclean knife or by falling on the road, it is advisable to take anti tetanus injection. If you are located at a place where anti tetanus injection is not available, one can take **6 pills of Ledum 200 as first aid**. Repeat the dose once a day for 3 days if anti tetanus injection is not accessible.

**Rabies**

If one is bitten by an unknown dog, monkey or any other animal, one must get a course of anti-rabies injection even if it means travelling to the nearest city. **6 pills of Ledum 200** should be taken as a part of first aid.

**Insomnia**

Insomnia or inability to sleep is a common problem. Homeopathy has many medicines for preventing insomnia. One dose of 6 pills of the medicine should be taken half an hour before going to sleep.

- **Insomnia of the aged:** Aconite 30
- **When over tired:** Arnica 200
- **Due to physical or mental restlessness:** Arsenic Alb 200
- **Sleepy but cannot sleep:** Cannabis Indica 30.
- **Due to pain:** Chamomilla 200.
- **In women after copious menstruation:** China 200
- **Due to mental activity:** Coffea Cruda 200
- **When you wake up at 3:00 AM:** Nux Vomica 200

**Cramps while Sleeping**

Cramp is a sudden involuntary contraction of a muscle or muscles. They cause severe pain. Cramps are of two types; those suffered by athletes and sportspersons due to over exertion or dehydrations and elderly persons while they sleep. The first kind can be prevented by taking rehydrating drinks at intervals during the sporting activity as permitted. The second category happens in almost one third of persons over 60. It is usually due to inadequate circulation of blood. This type of **cramps can be prevented by physiotherapy to improve blood circulation in lower extremities and by wearing compression stocking.** Unfortunately, wearing compression stocking is an ordeal by itself. **Grandpa has been able to reduce attacks of cramps in Grandma by administering Cuprum Ars 200 and Cuprum Met 200, one dose of six pills once or twice a week before going to sleep.**

**Prevention of Cancers**

Grandpa believes that cancers can be prevented. The factors which increase the risk of cancer are:

- **Radiation.** Exposure to nuclear radiation can cause cancer.
- **Sunlight.** Sunlight has ultraviolet rays which are harmful. Excessive exposure to sun, particularly between 9 AM and 4 PM can cause cancer.
- **Tobacco.** Smoking or chewing tobacco can cause cancer.
- **Cancer Causing Substances or Carcinogens.** These include pesticides, benzene, formaldehyde (used for preserving meat, fish and poultry), asbestos powder, stone dust, silicon dust, benzene, radon, cadmium, coal tar, nickel compounds, carbon soot, etc. People using carcinogens must take adequate precautions like wearing masks, gloves and wash their hands, faces and bodies if exposed. Purchase of fresh meat, fish and poultry is a must. Fish must be well washed in running water to remove carcinogens.
- **Chronic Inflations.** Sores, corns, boils, gum boils, blisters in the mouth etc if allowed to go uncured for a long time can cause cancer. Chronic infections of liver, kidney, lungs, intestines, uterus and colon are more difficult to detect. However, pain or discomfort in any of these organs must never be neglected. Pain or unusual bleeding in abdomen of women must be investigated and treated.
- **Processed Food.** Excessive use of processed food like corn beef, ham, sausages, charred meat, pasta etc, trans fats, etc can cause cancer. Unfortunately, working couples, single men and women and students often base their diet on processed food and fast food which are bad for health.
- **Alcohol.** Excessive drinking is likely to lead to liver damage and cancer.

- **Age, obesity and sedentary life.** These reduce the bodies resistance. Hence elderly and obese persons are more likely to suffer from cancer.

Grandpa says that we must take all possible precautions against the factors mentioned above. As far as possible avoid processed food. It is possible to cook great dishes like kababs, biriyani, etc using the "rice cooker" and "air fryer". Wear gloves, masks and protective goggles when working in toxic environments like spraying insecticides, paint etc. and when air quality is very poor. Peel all fruits and vegetables that can be pealed to avoid intake of residual pesticide. Scrape off charred portions of meat and bread.

**Grandpa also uses a dietary approach to prevent cancer.** He takes anti-oxidants in natural form as well as food supplements. Food which are rich in anti-oxidants and commonly available include apple, onions, egg plant or brinjal, beet, carrot, corn, kale, mangoes, pink grape fruit, pumpkin, sweet potatoes, tomatoes and water melon. Three major anti-oxidant vitamins are beta-carotene, vitamin C and vitamin E. In minerals, zinc and selenium are good anti-oxidants. Broccoli, cauliflower, cabbage, carrots, beans, berries, nuts, cinnamon, olive oil, turmeric, citrus foods, flax seeds, tomatoes, garlic and fatty fish are said to reduce chances of getting cancer and of cancer spreading.

**There is a vaccine for cervical cancer in women.** It is caused by a virus known as Human Papilloma Virus or HPV which is transmitted during unprotected sex. The vaccine is given to women aged between 13 and 26. Two doses six months apart is recommended and costs about Rs 6000 to Rs 8000.

**Uterine Cancer** is one of the most common types of cancer in women. Early symptoms are bleeding between menstrual cycles or after menopause. The risk can be reduced by maintaining a healthy weight and controlling diabetes. Some oral contraceptives can reduce risk. One should consult a competent doctor on this. If there are tumours in the uterus and the woman is past reproductive stage, it may be advisable to remove the uterus through surgery.

**Breast Cancer** is a common threat to women. The symptoms could be a lump in the breast or armpit, thickening or swelling of any part of the breast, irritation or redness, pulling in of nipples and pain or bleeding of nipples. All women must be alert to these problems and see a specialist as early as possible.

**Cancer of Mouth** is on the rise. Even if one has given up smoking or chewing tobacco, one needs to be very careful about oral health. Blisters or discolouring of the inside of the cheeks, blisters or redness on the edges of the tongue, changing colour of tongue to blue or black, painful cracks in the corner of lips and bleeding or painful gums and teeth must never be neglected. One must get these problems checked by a dentist and if the problem persists by a specialist. Grandpa believes that regularly washing the mouth before going to sleep with a mouth wash or 10 drops of Calendula Q in half a glass of tap water will reduce the chances of cancer of mouth. Taking Lyco Red capsules and applying Dologel to gums, lips and blisters in the mouth will further reduce the risk.

Grandpa also believes that **taking 6 pills of Arsenic Alb 1 M once a week** will reduce chances of cancer affecting any part of the body.

**Cancer is not incurable. With progress of medical science, the percentage of deaths from cancer has reduced considerably if detected early.** Grandpa's mother suspected she had breast cancer in 1992 when she was 63. She went for investigation. She was found positive and treated. She recovered and lived past 99. Early detection and treatment make all the difference. Cancer is not contagious. Negative mental attitude, taking artificial sweeteners, tumour biopsy, exposure to air, use of cell-phones, living near hi-tension lines do not cause cancer.

**Conclusion**

Homeopathy offers many options for prevention of diseases. However, **these should not be considered to be an alternative to allopathic immunization programs initiated by the Government but to supplement it.** This is particularly true for children.

The preventive medicines should not be taken unless there is a possibility of the problem occurring. Even after taking the medicine, one should continue to take recommended precautions to avoid infection. Some of the illnesses mentioned above are life threatening. **If symptoms occur even after taking the preventive medicine, one must see a doctor as early as possible.**

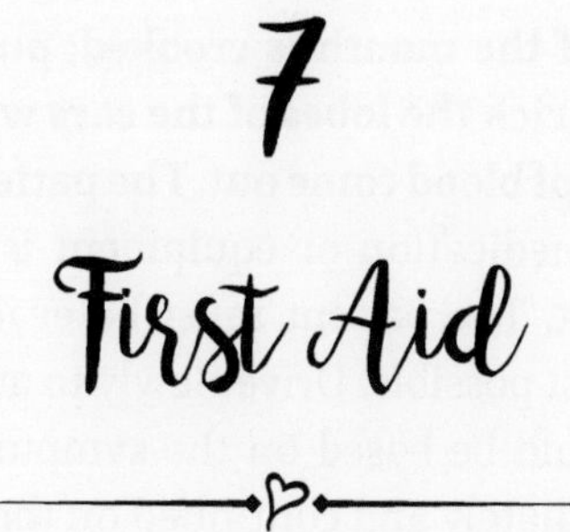

# 7 First Aid

Proper and timely first aid is often the difference between life and death. Homeopathy offers first aid not only in case of accidents or injuries but also for medical emergencies like heart attack, strokes, food poisoning etc. This chapter deals with emergencies and suggests use of homeopathic medicines for providing first aid. **It should be clear that every effort must be made, particularly in serious cases, to take the patient to a practicing doctor or hospital as early as possible. However, when ambulance with attendant is not available and effective medical aid cannot be reached within a few hours, it may be desirable to hold and treat the patient at a local hospital or medical centre till he is fit to take the rigors of the journey.** This is the fundamental philosophy in the Army's chain of evacuation of casualties. It is unfortunate but true that in many cases a patient dies because he is taken on a long journey to the hospital when he is not strong enough to undertake the journey. **If a patient has to be held at home for some time, he should be given whatever life-saving medicines are available, allopathic or homeopathic. Homeopathy has many life-saving treatments.**

**Apoplexy or Stroke**

**Apoplexy also called a stroke is a sudden, problem caused by bursting or blocking of a blood vessel of the brain.** There can be loss of consciousness, collapse and facial paralysis. It can be triggered in patients of high blood pressure due to extreme anger or emotional stress and accident. The patient should not be moved immediately. He should be helped to sit up wherever he is and prevented from falling over. **As per internet information, a simple procedure may prevent permanent disability and enable the patient to recover fast. Sterilize a needle or a pin with fire and prick all the ten finger tips of the hand till a drop of blood comes out of**

**each prick.** If blood does not come out squeeze the finger-tip to force the blood out. When blood starts oozing from the fingertips, the patient should regain consciousness. **If the mouth is crooked, pull the patients ears till they are red and then prick the lobes of the ears with the needle twice on each lobe till two drops of blood come out. The patient is expected to regain consciousness.** As no medication or equipment is involved, there should be no harm in trying it. The patient must be evacuated to a hospital by ambulance at the earliest possible. Drive slowly to avoid jerks.

The medication should be based on the symptoms as given below and should be started immediately and continued on the way to the hospital:

- **Right side facial paralysis with difficulty in reading and writing.** Dissolve 10 pills of Causticum 200 in a cup of water and administer one spoon of medicine every 15 minutes.
- **Left side facial paralysis with difficulty in reading and writing.** Dissolve 10 pills of Lachesis 200 in a cup of water and administer one spoon of medicine every 15 minutes.
- **If there is no facial paralysis, only redness and discomfort**, administer Belladonna 200 in the same way as described above.

**Appendicitis**

Appendicitis is an inflammation of the appendix, a small part in the right side of the lower abdomen. There is unbearable pain. Pain is worse on movement. There is also nausea, vomiting and foul breath. The disease is life threatening and immediate surgery is recommended to remove the appendix. **The patient should be given 6 pills of Belladonna 200 and 6 pills of Silicia 200 and taken to the hospital.**

**Asphyxiation**

**Asphyxiation is inadequate supply of oxygen to the lungs which in turn leads to inadequate supply of oxygen to the blood. It can lead to brain damage or death.** It can occur due to blocking of the throat by chocking due to food or liquid stuck in the throat or food pipe. It can also be due to accidents like children putting their head into plastic bags or sleeping in a closed room with a electric heater, kerosene lamp or candle. It can also result from an attack of Asthma or Bronchitis.

In case of choking due to food or liquid, effort should be made to clear the blockage by hard slaps on the back between the shoulders. If this does not work, make the patient lie face down with the stomach on one's lap and keep slapping as indicated earlier. Once the obstruction comes out, put the patient on his back and turn his head to one side. Clean the mouth with a piece of wet cloth. Dissolve 10 pills of Carbo Veg 200 in half a cup of water and give one teaspoon every half hour. Once the medicine finishes, give 6 pills of Carbo Veg 200 two times a day for a day or two. **The same medicine should be administered in cases of accidents with plastic bags or carbon monoxide poisoning. Serious patients should be evacuated to a hospital or nursing home where oxygen is available.**

**Asthma Attack**

**Severe Asthmatic attack can result in asphyxiation.** Persons with Asthma should have two types of inhalers prescribed by a doctor. One is preventive and should be taken morning and evening during change of season. The other, usually Asthelin, is SOS and is to be taken when there is wheezing. The patient should be made to sit in an upright position with the fore arm resting on some support like the back of a chair and elbows spread out so that there is no pressure on the chest. The room should be kept warm and moist by boiling some water in the room.

**If the inhaler is not available, dissolve 10 pills of Aconite 30 and Ipecac 200 in two separate half cups of water. One spoon of the medicines should be given to the patient alternately starting with Aconite every 15 minutes.** The solution of the medicine should be stirred each time before administering it. As soon as the attack is controlled, the patient can lie down and the interval of administering the medicine can be increased to one hour. **If the condition of the patient does not improve, evacuate to hospital or nursing home where oxygen is available as soon as possible.**

**Bleeding External**

**Try to stop the bleeding by pressing a clean handkerchief or any cloth on the wound. If no cloth is available, the wound should be pressed with hand to stop the flow.** If possible, raise the limb which is bleeding. Wash wound with Dettol or any available antiseptic. Dress the wound after the bleeding is controlled. Administer 10 pills of Arnica 1000 or 200 and Hamamelis 200 in that order. The medicines should be dissolved in two separate half cups of water. One spoon of the medicines should be given to the patient alternately starting with Arnica every 15 minutes. The solution of the medicine should be stirred each time before administering it. **As soon as the bleeding is controlled, the interval of administering the medicine can be increased to one hour till bleeding stops.** Apply Calendula mother tincture or ointment on the wound.

**Bleeding Internal**

**Internal bleeding can take place due to injuries and other reasons. It is difficult to detect until it is too late.** I know of two instances where accident victims, apparently without serious injuries, died due to internal bleeding. One was the victim of a vehicle accident. The other had fallen from the roof of a single storied structure. **As there are no symptoms of internal bleeding, it should be assumed whenever there is a suspected injury to the stomach or chest due to pressure or blow from a blunt instrument.** Administer 6 pills of Arnica 1000 or 200, Millefolium 200 and Hamamelis 200 in that order with 15 minutes gap between medicines as early as possible after an accident where internal injuries are suspected. Repeat dose after 4 hours.

**Burns and Scalds**

Burn injuries occur due to contact of skin with fire or extreme heat. Scalds take place due contact of the skin with hot liquids like boiling water or tea etc. Burns can also be chemical and occur when the skin comes in contact with corrosive chemicals like acids. **Burns or scalds or chemical burns should be washed with ice cold water containing Cantharis mother tincture.** Ice can also be applied. 6 pills of Hypericum 200 should be administered orally and Cantharis ointment or mother tincture should be gently applied on the damaged skin. Chemical burns should first be washed in cold running water for a few minutes before being treated the same way as ordinary burns and scalds. 6 pills of Cantharis 200 and Hypericum 200 should be administered two times a day for a few days till the wound begins to heal. **Blisters should never be punctured. In case of serious burns, one must see a doctor as early as possible. Burns can get infected if neglected. It is advisable to see a doctor and take anti- biotics.** If doctor is not accessible, add 6 pills of Arnica 200 to reduce chance of infection.

**Black Eye**

**Black eye occurs due to injury to the eye due to a blow or impact. The area around the eye turns black or dark blue due to internal bleeding.** Put ice or a wet cloth to the area. Administer 6 pills of Arnica 1000 and Ledum 200 alternately. Repeat after four hours.

**Coma**

A person can faint due to many reasons. Whatever the cause, the treatment is pour 5 drops of Camphor mother tincture on a teaspoon of sugar and hold it to the nose of the patient. This is to be repeated every 15 minutes till the patient regains consciousness.

**Concussion or Head Injury**

Concussion or head injury can occur due to fall from a two-wheeler, in a vehicle accident, due to fall from a height or due to some heavy object falling on the head. **It should be taken seriously even if the patient appears to be all right after the accident.** Administer 6 pills of Arnica 1000 or 200 and Hypericum 200. Repeat after four hours. Continue administering the medicines twice a day for 3 to 5 days. The patient should be made to rest and kept under observation and taken to a doctor if he shows any signs of discomfort or if the injury is feared to be serious.

**Cramps**

**An involuntary contraction of muscles which is very painful and can occur in the thigh, calves or feet while lying down or sleeping.** It can also occur in thighs, legs, hands, palms and fingers due to fatigue. To relieve the immediate pain, try to stretch the affected muscle. In case of cramps in the feet, the toes should be gently pulled outwards. In case of cramps of the thigh or calves, efforts should be made to straighten the knee and legs, if necessary, with assistance. For cramps in arms or palm, the fingers should be gently pulled outwards.

**For cramps in calves, soles of feet and palms,** take 6 pills of Cuprum Met 200 or Cuprum Ars 200. **In case of cramps in fingers or palm due to strain** take Ruta G 200. The patient should also take one packet of oral re-hydration medicine dissolved in water or a few glasses of water containing one pinch of salt and one teaspoon of sugar.

**Cuts or Punctured Wounds**

Cuts from knives, glass or any other item should first be cleaned thoroughly with an antiseptic solution. Apply Calendula mother tincture or ointment. **Take one dose of Arnica 1000 and Hypericum 200 to reduce pain and two doses of Ledum 200 at 4 hr interval. In case of punctured wounds caused by nail or thorn, take two doses of Ledum 200 at 4 hours interval.**

**Dog Bites**

Dog bite should be considered to be a punctured wound and treated as indicated above. However, give one dose of Arnica 1000 immediately to relieve mental shock. Clean the wound with hot water and antiseptics and apply Calendula mother tincture or ointment. **See a doctor and take anti rabies injections if available. If anti-rabies injection is not available, take 6 pills of Ledum 200 twice a day for three days.**

**Ear Ache**

Ear ache can be due to various reasons. Take a suitable painkiller and head to a doctor. Suggested Homeopathic medicines are as under:

- **Pain due to exposure to cold ai**r. One dose of Aconite 30 every hour till pain subsides.
- **Sudden terrible pain in middle or external ear.** Dissolve 10 pills of Belladona 200 in one cup of water and administer one tea spoon of the liquid once every 15 minutes. Increase interval as the pain reduces.
- **Due to boil or pus.** Myristica 200 or Silicea 200 one dose of 4 pills three times a day.
- **Along with toothache.** One dose of Plantago 30 every hour. Increase interval as pain reduces. Use Silicea 200 if Plantago is not available.

**Encephalitis**

**It is an acute and life-threatening viral infection which is common during monsoons in many parts of India. The patient has fever, headache, great body pain and stiffness all over the body. Take patient to hospital if available.** If there is an epidemic in the area and the symptoms are seen in anyone, dissolve 10 pills of Gelsemium 200 and Baptista 30 in two half cups of water and administer one teaspoon of the medicine alternately every half hour. The administration of Baptista 30 should continue in the same way. Gelsemium 200 should be administered two to three times a day till cured.

**Epileptic Fits**

**No effort should be made to control the movements of the affected person except to ensure that the person does not get hurt by striking against furniture or hard objects.** Dissolve 10 pills of Cuprum Met 200 in half a cup of water and administer one spoon of the liquid once every 15 minutes till the patient calms down. If the patient faints, treat him as indicated for Coma above. If the patient gets violent, moans or howls during attack and limbs cannot be straightened dissolve 10 pills of Cicuta 200 in half a cup of water and alternate with Cuprum Met till the patient stabilizes.

**Food Poisoning**

**The symptoms of food poisoning are repeated loose motion, stomach pain and vomiting within a short period after taking a meal. Give one does of Arsenic Alb 200 and head to a hospital.** If doctor or hospital is not available, give **one dose of Arsenic Alb 200 should be given once an hour till the symptoms stops.** It should be ensured that the patient does not get dehydrated by giving him glass full of "Electrol" oral re-hydration packet dissolved in one litre of water. If not available, give a solution of once pinch of salt and one teaspoon of sugar or glucose in one glass of water, once every hour. If the patient faints, treat him as indicated for Coma above.

**Foreign Bodies**

Sometimes foreign bodies like pieces of thorns, wood splinters or even sewing needle may get embedded in the skin and cannot be removed. **Sometimes fish bones may get stuck inside the mouth or throat.** Such foreign bodies can be removed by one dose of Silicea 200. Some times a second or third dose may be given after every four hours.

**Fracture**

Fractures occur due to pressure or a blow on a bone mostly due to accidents or falls. A bone may be dislocated, cracked or broken into two or more pieces. Sometimes broken bone pierces the skin and is visible. Pain is very severe and the person is unable to move the extremities of the broken part. The fractured portion should be immobilized with splints and surgical or crepe bandage. A sling to support the arm should be used if the injury is to the collar bone, shoulder, arm, wrist or fingers. In case of injuries to hip, thigh, leg or feet, the patient should only be move on a stretcher or a wheel chair. **Dissolve 10 pills of Arnica 1000 and Ruta 200 in two half cups of water and administer one spoonful of the liquid alternately every 15 minutes till the pain is bearable. Another medicine very useful in treating injuries to bones and reducing pain is Symphytom 30. Take the patient to an orthopaedic surgeon for setting the bone as soon as possible.**

**Frostbite**

In sub-zero temperatures, exposed parts or parts without adequate blood circulation like toes, finger, nose, chin, cheek and lobes of the ears may develop paleness, numbness and blisters. **If severe, the affected portion may develop gangrene.** The patient should be removed from the freezing conditions. **Direct heat must never be applied to the affected part. The part should be gently messaged with hand till circulation of the blood restarts.** Rhus Ven mother tincture or Rhus Ven 30 in liquid form should be applied on the affected part which should then be covered with soft cloth or surgical cotton and lightly bandaged. **The patient should be evacuated to a warmer shelter as early as possible.** Agaricus 30 should be given three times a day till recovery to reduce burning, itching and swelling. If there are signs of gangrene like foul smell, give Hepar Sulf 200 four times a day till recovery. If the patient is diabetic, give Arsenic Alb 200 in place of Hepar Sulph 200.

**Heart Attack**

Symptoms of heart attack are severe constricting pain in the chest and or in the left arm upwards to the neck. There is cold sweating and difficulty in breathing. Pulse is weak and irregular. Sometimes, the patient may lose consciousness. The patient must lie down on his back wherever he is. Clothing round neck and waist should be loosened. If unconscious, artificial respiration can be started. **If Solbitrate is available, place one pill below the tongue. Also dissolve two tablets of Dispirin and feed the patient with it with a spoon. Give one dose of Arnica 1000 immediately and repeat after every hour.** Mix 10 drops of Cactus mother tincture in half a cup of water and administer one teaspoon of the liquid every 15 minutes till the condition stabilizes. If there is loss of consciousness, try to revive by procedure given under Coma above.

***Do not attempt to move the patient to a hospital till the condition stabilizes. Call ambulance with necessary equipment.***

**Heat Stroke**

**Long exposure to severe heat (above 45 degrees centigrade) can result in heat stroke. The patient is thirsty, feels dizzy and exhausted. He has headache, nausea and feels drowsy. The patient may also have loose motions. Dehydration can occur. The body temperature rises above 104 degrees Fahrenheit or 40 degrees Centigrade. The patient may become unconscious and die.**

The patient should be wrapped in wet cloth and moved to a cool room or air-conditioned room. Make the patient drink substantial quantities of water mixed with salt and sugar or fruit juices. Use cold compress with cloth soaked in ice cold water. Give one dose of Glonoine 200 three times a day. The first dose may be dissolved in half a cup of water to make administration of medicine easier. ***Persons traveling or working in extreme heat should carry a dram of Glonoine 200 pills in their pocket and take a dose if they feel uncomfortable.***

**Injury to Back or Neck**

**Severe back or neck injury can result in paralysis. The patient should not be moved except on a stretcher or ambulance.** One dose of Arnica 1000 should be administered immediately and continued thrice a day till condition stabilizes. Hypericum 200 should be administered immediately after Arnica and continued three times a day till the condition stabilizes.

**Injury to Eye**

Injury to eye can be due to a blow, foreign body or chemical burn. In case of physical injury administer one dose of Arnica 1000 and continue twice a day till cured. Incase of foreign body like sand or insect, remove foreign body with a piece of clean soft cloth and administer one dose of Arnica 1000. In case of chemical burn, wash the eye thoroughly with a jug of cold water mixed with 10 drops of Cantharis mother. **Take to an eye hospital immediately after first aid.**

**Injury to Nerves**

**The nerves in fingers can be injured due to a hammer blow or due to a door or window closing on it. Nerves in the tail bone may be hurt due to a fall. These injuries are extremely painful.** One dose of Arnica 1000 should be administered immediately and continued twice a day till condition stabilizes. Hypericum 200 should be administered half hour after Arnica and continued three to four times a day till the pain subsides. **One should take patient to a hospital as early as possible and get an x-ray or scan done.**

**Insect Bites and Stings**

Immediately give one dose of Apis 1000. If there is a punctured wound which bleeds scantily give one dose of Ledum 200. Repeat Apis if necessary, after 4 hours.

**Pain**

**Severe pain cries for relief. Over the counter analgesics if available should be administered immediately if available but not on empty stomach.** Some suggested Homeopathic medicines are given below. One dose should be given immediately and repeated every three to four hours.

- **Sudden violent pain due to exposure to cold air.** Aconite 30.
- **Pain due to injury to nerves of fingers, toes, nails, crushed finger tips or tail bone.** Arnica 1000 and Hypericum 200.
- **Severe pain in muscles.** Calcarea Carb 30.
- **Pain in bones.** Eupator Perf 200.
- **Pain in wrist or fingers or eyes due to over use.** Ruta G 200

**Shock**

**Shock is a mental state in a person when he or she is unable to think and behave rationally. It can be due to accidents with or without injury and emotional trauma due to death of a spouse or children, discovery of infidelity in spouse or crippling financial loss.** Try to make the patient as physically comfortable as possible. Mix 10 pills of Arnica 1000 and Aconite 30 in two separate cups of water and administer one spoon of the liquid alternately every 30 minutes. Repeat after the medicine finishes. The interval between medicines can be gradually increased after the first few hours.

**Snake Bite**

Apply tourniquet if the bite is on a leg or hand to stop the poison from spreading. Give a dose of Arnica 1000 immediately to relieve mental shock and a dose of Aconite 30 to reduce fear of death. Try to suck or squeeze out some blood from the wound to reduce poison in the body. Thereafter **give alternate doses of Lachesis 200 and Arsenic Alb 200 every 4 hours till you can reach a doctor**. Apply hot fomentation to the area around the bite.

**Sprains and Strains**

Sprains may occur at joints due to injury or excessive use. It may also be caused by lifting or trying to lift heavy weights from an incorrect posture. Ankles, wrists, elbows, hips, knees or shoulders are most likely to be affected. **Put some ice in a polythene bag and give cold compress to the affected part. Do not massage.** If the sprain is due to injury, give alternate doses of Arnica 1000 and Ruta G 200 every four hours. If there is only strain, give 4 pills of Ruta 200 three times a day. **If the pain is unbearable, give allopathic painkillers, pills, sprays and ointments, along with the Homeopathic medicines.**

**Conclusion**

Emergencies can occur at any time during day or night. Medical assistance may not be immediately available. Some injuries or attacks are not life threatening. At other times, the patient may not be in a fit condition to move. In such cases, Homeopathy offers simple first aid solutions which relieve pain and save lives. **It is however important to remember that first aid is for immediate relief and not always a total cure. See a doctor, Allopathic, Homeopathic or Ayurvedic or a dentist as early as possible and get totally cured.**

# 8

# Problems of Mind, Head and Fevers

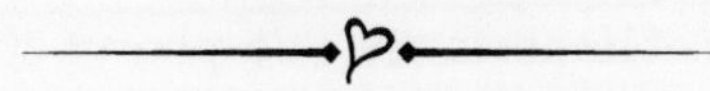

**Alcoholism**

Some symptoms and medicines to be taken two times a day are given below. If they do not work, the only option may me taking the person to a re-habitation centre.

- **Excessive Desire for Alcohol.** Drinking leads to vomiting. Arsenic Alb 200. Continue till habit is reduced.
- **Fond of drinking, rich food and women.** Sleeps late and wakes up with hangover. Wakes up with nausea. Best remedy for one who has taken a peg too many. Nux Vomica 200.
- **Chronic alcoholism.** Eats little. Sulphuric Acid 30. Continue for a month. Another medicine that can be tried is Avena Sativa Q, 20 drops in warm water thrice daily. **If the patient is unwilling to undergo treatment, the medicine can be mixed in the normal water he drinks.**

**Amnesia or Memory loss**

Amnesia means loss of memory. It can be due to head injury, alcoholism, and epilepsy or brain tumour. It can also be due to emotional shock. **The primary medicine is Anacardium 200. The dosage should be 4 No 20 pills three to four times a day.** If the loss of memory is due to emotional shock, the treatment should be started with Arnica 1000. Dissolve ten pills of Arnica 1000 in half a cup of lukewarm water. Administer one tea spoon of the liquid every half hour. Start Anacardium 15 minutes after the second dose of Arnica. Some symptoms and medicines to be taken two times a day are given below:

- **Loss of memory and self-confidence.** Dementia in old age. Aversion to strangers. Childish. Grieves over trifles. Baryta Carb 200.
- **Forgetful, confused and low spirited. Anxiety with palpitation. Obstinacy and aversion to exertion.** Calcarea Carb 200.
- **Very forgetful. Cannot finish sentences. Cannot remember one's identity**. Canibis Indica 200.
- **Weak memory. Cannot find the right word. Apathic. Indifferent to surroundings.** Acid Phosphoric 200.
- **Loss of memory. Hyper sensitive. Afraid of death when alone. Exaggerated feeling of importance.** Phosphorus 200.
- **Inability to recall or remember recent events.** Absinthium 30.
- **Due to injury.** Arnica 1000.
- **Forgets names of well-known streets, house or persons.** Sulphur 200 and Glonoine 200

**Apathy or Indifference to Everything**

Some symptoms and medicines to be taken two times a day are given below:

- **Clumsy. Drops things easily. Jealous, fidgety and hard to please. Complains and cribs all the time.** Apis 200.
- **Disobedient, taciturn and despondent. Disposition to hurt others feelings.** China Off 200. **If the person does not want treatment, take the medicine in liquid form and mix 10 drops in his water glass.**
- **Desires to be left alone. Apathy regarding one's illness.** Gelsemium 200.
- **Apathy caused by grief or mental shock. Delirium and despair**. Acid Phosphoric 200.
- **Melancholic, sad and tearful. Non communicative. Keeps sighing and sobbing.** Ignatia 200.
- **Indifferent to loved ones and family. Easily offended. Dreads to be alone. Very sad. Miserly.** Sepia 200. **If the person does not want treatment, take the medicine in liquid form and mix 10 drops in his water glass.**

**Depression, Fear and Anxiety**

Some common symptoms and medicines which are to be taken two times a day are given below:

- **Great fear of death and everything without any reason.** Aconite 30
- **Disgusted with life. Talks of committing suicide.** Aurum Met 200. Do not leave the person alone. Discuss the persons problem and try to cheer the person up. Sweating it out by playing a game or going for a walk canhelp.
- **Mental depression. Thinks only of death and salvation.** Graphites 200.
- **Melancholic depression with loss of self-confidence. Afraid to be left alone.** Lycopodium 200 and Phosphorous 200.
- **Depression on account of suffering from chronic diseases.** Carbo Veg 200 and Nat Mur 200.
- **Fear of failure or anxiety about journeys or events.** Argentum Nit 200.
- **Anxiety felt in the stomach.** Arsenic Alb 200 and Pulsatilla 30.

**Exhaustion or Debility**

Some common symptoms and medicines which are to be taken two times a day are given below:

- **In physically weak persons.** Alfalfa mother tincture 10 drops or Alfalfa tonic two times a day. Improves digestion. Increases body fat, weight, mental and physical vigour.
- **Exhaustion from slightest exertion or asthma, typhoid, malaria or at night.** Arsenic Alb 200.
- **Due to over work.** Calcarea Carb 200.
- **Due to chronic indigestion or acidity. Tiredness even from a short walk.** Carbo Veg 200 for four months.
- **Due to loss of body fluids or blood.** China 200.
- **Exhaustion of mind first and then body, nervous exhaustion, cannot collect thought.** Phosphoric Acid 30.
- **Due to over use of drugs, medicines or alcoholic drinks.** Nux Vomica 200.

**Hallucination**

Hallucination is seeing events which have never taken place. It is a brain disorder. Some common symptoms and medicines which are to be taken two times a day are given below:

- **Frightful visions with loss of memory of recent events.** Absinthium 30.
- **Patient thinks he is possessed by two persons.** Anacardium 200.
- **Visual hallucinations.** The patient sees ghosts, monsters, insects, animals etc which are out to hurt him. Belladonna 200.

**Hysteria**

**Hysteria is an irrational, uncontrollable, violent outburst of emotion or fear.** It is more common among women than men. Dissolve 10 pills of Ignatia 200 and Nat Mur 200 in half cups of water and administer one teaspoon of the liquid alternately every half an hour till the condition stabilizes. Thereafter, give two doses of 6 pills of Ignatia 200 for a week. **If the patient sings and laughs and suddenly changes from hilarity to melancholy** give two doses Crocus Savitus 30 for a week.

**Insomnia**

**Insomnia is a chronic inability to sleep or get adequate sleep.** Sleeping pills should be avoided. However, **some doctors prescribe Clonazepam Tablets 0.5 mg to be taken on a regular basis**. Listening to music or two small pegs of whiskey or wine can help. Some common symptoms and Homeopathic medicines which are to be taken two times a day for a week is given below:

- **Of the aged.** Aconite Nap 30.
- **Due to worry. Need to get up.** Ambra Grisea 30.
- **When physically over tired.** Arnica 200.
- **On account of physical or mental restlessness.** Arsenic Alb 200.
- **Sleepy but cannot sleep.** Canibis Indica 30.
- **Due to pain.** Chamomilla 200.
- **Due to mental activity, sorrow or joy, emotional excitement etc.** Coffea Cruda 200.
- Wakes up at 3.00 AM and goes back to sleep at 5.00 AM and wakes up feeling miserable. Nux Vomica 200.
- In women due to sexual desire. Raphanus 30.

**Irritable**

Some common symptoms and medicines which are to be taken two times a day for a week is given below:

- **Morose, irritable with "let me be alone attitude".** Arnica 200

- **Anxious, sad and irritable with suicidal tendencies.** Aurum Met 200 and Arsenic Alb 200.
- **Irritable due to body ache. Dislikes physical activity.** Bryonia 200.
- **Given to late nights and excessive drinking but extremely irritable, sullen and fault finding when not indulging himself.** Nux Vomica 200.
- **Violent temper.** Throws things, shouts, uses abusive language when angry. Tarantula Hispanica 30. **One dose of 10 drops of the medicine in liquid form mixes in the persons drinking water can cure him.**

**Mania**

Mania is a kind of insanity where a person displays strong desires or unacceptable behavior. Some common symptoms and medicines which are to be taken two times a day for a week is given below:

- **Must move continually. Cannot be Still.** Canibis Indica 30.
- **Sexual Mania. Fiery, unquenchable desire for sex.** Cantharis 200 and Phosphorous 200. Wives tired of sex may obtain the medicines in liquid form and mix 10 drops in drinking water of their husbands.
- **Tendency to indulge in obscene acts, gestures and expression**, Hyoscyamus 200.
- **Imagines being the subject of divine wrath.** Kali Bromatum 30.
- **Believes he is in communication with God and is carrying out God's commands**. Lachesis 200 and Stramonium 200
- **Unclean habits. Does nothing but meditating.** Sulphur 200.
- **Talks lewd.** Veratrum Alb 200.

**Melancholy, Pessimist**

Some common symptoms and medicines which are to be taken two times a day for a week is given below:

- **Weary and low spirited but obstinate and forgetful. Cannot cope with sustained mental activity.** Calcarea Carb 200.
- **Indifferent to happiness or sorrow. Crushed by prolonged illness.** Carbo Veg 200 and Nitric Acid 200.
- **Overburdened, harassed, exhausted housewife.** Sepia 200.

**Nightmares**

Some common symptoms and medicines which are to be taken two times a day for a week is given below:

- **Terrifying dreams which result in waking up.** Calcarea Carb 30.
- **Talking in sleep.** Hyoscyamus 200.

**Vertigo**

**Vertigo is the sensation of spinning in the head. The patient loses balance and falls.** Some common symptoms and medicines which are to be taken two times a day for a week is given below:

- **With tendency to fall backwards.** Absinthium 200.
- **On rising from bed.** Aconite 30.
- **From walking in the sun.** Agaricus 200 and Glonoine 200.
- **When going upstairs** Arsenic Hydro 30
- **When going down stairs.** Borax 200.
- **On seeing running water.** Ferrum Met 30.
- **With nausea and vomiting.** Ipecac 30
- **When climbing mountains.** Coca 30.
- **Looking down.** Phosphorus 200
- **Looking up.** Silicia 200.

**Apoplexy or Stroke**

After first aid has been administered and the patient has survived the attack, the patient may be in different conditions. These conditions and suggested medicines are given below:

- **Paralysis of left side of face, left arm and left leg.** 6 pills of Allium Cepa 200 two times a day till cured.
- **Paralysis of right side of face, right arm and right leg.** 6 pills of Causticum 200 two times a day till cured.
- **If patient does not recover from coma or jaws droop.** 4 pills of Opium 1000 once a week. If there is one sided paralysis add medicine as indicated above.

**Hair Problems**

Some common symptoms and medicines which are to be taken two times a day are given below:

- **Baldness.** Fluoric Acid 30. Take for a month.
- **Hair fall.** Phosphoric Acid 200 and Thuja 200. Take for a week. **Grandma uses Allen's Arnica Hair Root Vitalizer when having the problem and gets great results.**
- **Hair falls in large bunches.** Phosphorous 200. Take for a week.
- **Premature greying of hair.** Phosphoric Acid 200. Take for a month.

**Scalp Problems**

Some common symptoms and medicines which are to be taken two times a day for a week is given below:

- **Severe itching with dandruff. Cannot brush hair. Aggravation at night** Arsenic Alb 200 and Phosphorus 200.
- **Eczema on bald patches.** Lycopodium 200.

**Thrombosis**

**Thrombosis is blocking of an artery or vein due to a blood clot.** If in the brain it can lead to a stroke and has been discussed under stroke. If in the arteries leading to the heart, it can result in a heart attack also discussed under emergencies. **If the clot occurs in other regions, there is severe pain and even paralysis.** One can take Ecospirin 150, a blood thinner, which may dissolve the clot. **It is a serious medical problem and one must see a specialist as early as possible.**

Some medicines to be taken two times a day for a week are:

- **One sided paralysis with loss of speech.** Bothrops 30.
- **Paralysis or severe pain in extremities.** Merc Sol 200.

**Influenza or Flu**

**It is an infective viral disease.** It is advisable to wear a mask when in indoor confined spaces like air crafts, air ports, railway stations, shopping malls etc. In open areas try to maintain two metre social distancing. Start taking Paracetamol and Vitamin C tablets if you have body pain or sneezing and running nose. Add a cough syrup if you have a sore throat. **Get yourself tested for COVID 19, Dengue and Chikungunya if there an epidemic of the same in the area.**

Homeopathy treatment consists of one dose of Influenzin 200 daily. Administer a second medicine as suggested below two times a day till cured.

Paracetamol and Vitamin C can continue.

- **When there is cold and running nose or spittoon.** Arsenic Alb 200.
- **With bronchial problems.** Bryonia 200.
- **With pain in bones.** Eupatorium Perf 200.
- **With high temperature, pain in muscles.** Gelsemium 200.
- **At change of seasons.** Rhus Tox 200.

**Chills**

Some fevers are accompanied by cold and shaking of the body. The patient wants to be covered with blankets or quilts. Such fevers could be malaria or typhoid. A doctor must be seen and blood test carried out.

Some common symptoms and Homeopathic medicines which are to be taken two times a day are given below:

- **Fever with chill starting at 2.00 AM.** Calcarea Carb 200.
- **Periodic chills. Same time every day.** China 200.
- **Fever with chill, shivering and body pain.** Gelsemium 200.
- **Fever with chill that comes at 10.30 AM.** Nat Mur 200.
- **Chilliness in a warm room. Patient has no thirst.** Pulsatilla 30.

**Encephalitis**

**It is an acute and life-threatening viral infection which is common during monsoons in many parts of India.** It is more common among children than adults. The patient has fever, headache, great body pain and stiffness all over the body. Take the patient to the hospital as soon as possible.

If **there is an epidemic in the area, dissolve 10 pills of Gelsemium 200 and Baptista 30 in two half cups of water and administer one teaspoon of the medicine alternately every half hour as interim treatment. The administration of Baptista 30 should continue in the same way. Gelsemium 200 should be administered two times a day till cured.**

**Fever due to Exposure**

Some common symptoms and medicines which are to be taken two times a day are given below:

- **Fever due to exposure to cold.** Aconite 30.
- **Fever due to exposure to heat.** Glonoine 200.

- **Fever due to exposure to wet weather**. Dulcamara 200.
- **High fever with or without delirium. Cool with ice pack or wet cloth.** Belladonna 200.

**Intermittent/ Periodic Fever**

**Such fevers are likely to be malaria or typhoid. Both diseases are serious and life threatening. The patient must be taken to a doctor at the earliest.** In the interim give one dose of Arsenic Alb 200 and China 200 alternately, two times a day.

**Meningitis**

Meningitis is caused by a bacterial infection that can be life threatening. The patient should be taken to the hospital as early as possible. The onset can be sudden or gradual. There is severe headache and high fever. The neck or back is stiff and painful. There can be vomiting and convulsions. Symptoms and medicines are given below. The treatment should be started with Tuberculinum 200 if available. Other medicines should be started after six hours.

- **The patient cries of pain in sleep (delirium).** Apis 200.
- **Sudden onset with high temperatures, delirium, headache and photophobia.** Belladonna 200.
- **With convulsions, distortion of limbs and loss of consciousness.** Cicuta 200.
- **With nausea, vomiting, violent convulsions and pain in brain and eyes.** Cuprum Met 200.

# 9

# Problems of Eyes, Ears, Nose, Mouth, Teeth and Throat

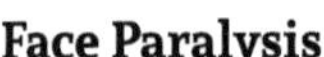

**Face Paralysis**

In this case there is paralysis of the face only. The patient should be taken to a doctor. Sometimes saliva may dribble from the corner of the mouth. Some suggested medicines to be given twice a day till cured are:

- **Sudden attack due to exposure to cold air.** Aconite 30
- **Left sided affected.** Lachesis 200
- **Right side affected.** Causticum 200
- **Facial muscles around moth contracted, eyes cannot close.** Gelsemium 200.
- **Distortion of facial muscles with twitching of the corners of the mouth.** Opium 200.

**Blindness**

Sudden attacks of blindness or blurred vision can occur due to retina related problems. Some medicines, to be taken two times a day, are:

- **Day blindness.** Bothrops 30
- **Colour blindness.** Carbo Sulf 30.
- **Night blindness in anaemic patients or during menses.** China 200.
- **Letters move during reading, lines disappear.** Cicuta 200

**Burning in Eyes**

If there is a burning sensation in the eye, take 6 pills of Allum Cepa 200 and Arsenic Alb 200, two times a day till the problem is cured.

**Cataract**

Cataract is a common problem in the aged. **Surgery is usually necessary to replace the lens. One must go to an eye specialist who does such operations every day. Only one eye should be operated at a time.** One dose of Arnica 1000 should be taken before the operation. These operations are not always successful. Grandpa's father lost eyesight in both eyes after cataract operations. **After operation care is very important and precautions recommended by the doctor must be taken faithfully.**

If detected in early stages, treatment under Homeopathy is possible. **Cineraria Homeopathic eye drops are said to cure cataract and corneal opacity without surgery. It is used externally, one drop in each eye three times a day for six months. Stop if there is excessive pain or burning after giving drops.** Progress must be monitored and surgery should be done if adequate improvement is not seen.

Some symptoms and medicines are as under. **Start treatment with one dose of Sulphur 200. No other medicines that day.**

- **Vision is foggy. Eyes water. Worse in the morning.** Calcarea Carb 200.
- **In early stages, when there is severe myopia (short sightedness).** Give one dose of Causticum 1000 once a week.
- **Soft cataract. Not ready for surgery. Vision is hazy.** Naphthalene 30.
- **Cataract with photophobia (intolerance of bright light). Black spots appear before eyes. Printed letters appear red.** Phosphorous 200.

**Conjunctivitis**

**Conjunctivitis is inflammation of a membrane which covers the white of the eye. The eyes turn red. There is a feeling of sand in the eye. The eyelids are swollen. The eye becomes sensitive to light. The disease is infective.** The medicines to be taken two times a day till cured are:

- **Stinging pain and watering eyes.** Apis 1000.
- **Watering eyes but no pain.** Arg Nit 200.
- **Sudden attack and no discharge from eye.** Belladona 200.
- **Shooting pain in bones above the eye, discharge and pus.** Hepar Sulph 200.

### Detached Retina

**Detached retina is a serious problem which requires immediate medical attention of an eye specialist as early as possible.** Patient sees flashes of light in the corner of the eye. If unattended may lead to sudden painless loss of vision. The patient should lie down and rest and must avoid jerks. Symptoms and medicines to be taken as an interim measure are:

- **Upper half of vision curtained, lower clear.** One dose of Aurum Met 200 and Naphthalene 30 two times a day.
- **Caused by injury Arnica 1000.** One dose two times a day.
- **Double vision and dark spots.** One dose of Gelsemium 200 and Naphthalene 30 two times a day

### Double vision

Some common symptoms and medicines which are to be taken two times a day are given below:

- **Double vision when seeing with one or both eyes.** Gelsemium 200.
- **Sees double with both eyes but normal with one eye.** Plumbum Met 30
- **When objects appear with coloured borders.** Hyoscyamus 200

### Eye Lashes

Some common problems and medicines which are to be taken two times a day are given below:

- **Turned inwards.** Borax 200
- **Drooping eyelids.** Conium 200.
- **Loss of eyelashes.** Petroleum 30.

### Glaucoma

**This is a serious problem and requires specialist medical attention at the earliest.** The patient has progressive loss of vision due to increased pressure inside the eyeball. There is acute pain and blurring of vision. The severe pain may cause vomiting. The interim medicines are:

- **With pain and rainbow like or green halo around lights.** One dose of Osmium 30 two times a day.

- **Objects look red or blue. Sometimes there is momentary blindness.** One dose of Phosphorous 200 two times a day.

**Itching in Eyes**

Some common symptoms and medicines which are to be taken two times a day are given below:

- **Itching of eyeballs.** Ambrosia 200
- **Itching of area inside the eyelids.** Zincum Met 200.

**Stye**

**A stye is a pimple on the eye lid which can be filled with pus.** Give one dose of Pulsatilla 30 two times a day. If there is excessive swelling of eye lids also give Apis 1000 two times a day.

**Twitching in Eye**

In case of continuous twitching of eyelids or eyeballs, give Agaricus 200 two times a day.

**Watering of Eyes**

Some common symptoms and medicines which are to be taken two times a day are given below:

- **Copious flow with itching of eyelids.** Ambrosia 30.
- **Copious flow with burning and swelling of eye lids.** Euphrasia 200.
- **With inflamed eyelids glued together with yellow discharge.** Pulsatilla 30.

**Nose Bleeding**

Some symptoms and suggested medicines to be given two times a day are given below:

- **Daily attacks in weak persons.** Carbo Veg 200.
- **Small quantities with nasal discharge.** Phosphorous 200.
- **Bleeding when hard crust in nose is loosened.** Silecia 200.

**Pain in Nose**

**When there is pain in nasal bones with swelling,** take 6 pills of Merc Sol 200 two times a day.

**Polyps in Nose**

**Polyps are a small growth in the nose.** Suggested medicines to be taken two times a day are:

- **At the base of the nose with foul smell.** Calcarea Carb 200.
- **With bleeding.** Phosphorous 200.

**Running Nose**

Some common symptoms and medicines which are to be taken two times a day are given below:

- **With violent sneezing. Eyes water profusely.** Allium Cepa 200.
- **Sudden violent attack. Itching of eyelids.** Ambrosia 30.
- **Thin watery discharge. Burning sensation. Patient restless. Better from hot drinks, worse from cold drinks.** Arsenic Alb 200.
- **Thick, string like, yellow-green inward discharge comes out as sputum.** Kali Bi 200.
- **Yellow, green and thick.** Merc Sol 200 and Pulsatilla 30.

**Sinusitis**

**Sinusitis is infection in sinuses or cavities in bones leading from skull to the nose. Pain is worse when stooping down, lying down or coughing.** Mucus which can be green, yellow, grey or mixed is discharged outwards through the nose or inwards into the throat. Nose is blocked. Take one dose of Hepar Sulph 200 and Kali Iod 30 two times a day till cured.

**Sneezing**

The symptoms and suggested medicines to be taken two times a day till cured are:

- **Cold starts with sneezing and running nose.** Nat Mur 200.
- **Due to exposure to cold.** Aconite 30
- **Continuous without relief.** Arsenic Alb 200.

**Loss of Hearing**

Loss of hearing can be due to aging or other causes. The under mentioned medicines should be taken two times a day till cured:

- **Hardness of hearing. Crackling sound in ear. Glands around ears swollen.** Baryta Carb 200.

- **Due to water getting into ear. Pain may be there.** Calcarea Carb 200
- **With fetid pus coming out of the ear.** Silecia 200. Can be taken with the medicines mentioned above.
- **With whizzing and throbbing in the ear.** Hepar Sulph 200.
- **With eczema or if hears better in noise.** Graphite 200. Calendula mother tincture should be applied to the ear with ear buds.
- **Loss of hearing due to wax in the ear.** Conium 200.
- **With violent roaring and buzzing.** Carbo Sulph 30 and Chininum Sulph 30
- **Loss of hearing due to aging.** Pulsatilla 30 and Phosphorus 200.

**Noises in Ears**

**Sometimes one can hear funny noises even when there is no external source of the noise.** Symptoms with medicines to be taken two times a day are:

- **Ringing, roaring or buzzing sound in the ear when chewing, swallowing or sneezing.** Baryta Mur 30
- **Hears own echo.** Causticum 200
- **Ringing, roaring or buzzing sound when suffering from cold.** Kali Mur 30.
- **Sound of bells ringing.** Ledum 200
- **Roaring or pistol like sound along with discharge of pus.** Silicia 200.

**Paralysis of Tongue**

Tongue is black and paralyzed. There is frothing in the mouth. See a doctor at the earliest. Take one dose of Opium 200 two times a day till cured.

**Problems of the Lips**

Some common problems of lips and mouth and their medicines are given below. 6 pills of the medicine should be taken two times a day till cured.

- **Cracks at the corner of the mouth.** Antim Crud 200 and Borax 200.
- **Lips swollen due to any reason including insect bite.** Apis Mel 200.
- **Lips black.** Arsenic Alb 200
- **Lips dry and cracked.** Bryonia 200
- **Lips pain when touched.** Hepar Sulph 200.
- **Lips cracked during winter.** Petroleum 200.

**Problems of the Tongue**

Some common problems of the tongue and their medicines are given below. 6 pills of the medicine should be taken two times a day till the problems are cured.

- **Thick milky white coating.** Antim Crud 200
- **Swollen and fiery red.** Apis 1000
- **Blue and ulcerated.** Arsenic Alb 200.
- **Covered with blisters.** Merc Sol 200 and Carbo Veg 200
- **Constant protrusion and retraction.** Cuprum Met 200
- **White blisters on the edge.** Thuja 200

**Stammering**

Some common symptoms and medicines which are to be taken two times a day are given below:

- **Stammering in a person with awkward movements. Things keep falling from the hand.** Bovista 30.
- **Stammering with repetition of initial consonants. There is hesitation and confusion.** Cannabis Sativa 30.
- **Due to fear, particularly in young girls.** Pulsatilla 30.

**Teeth**

**Serious problems of the teeth which are the result of long years of neglect of oral health like dental cavities or crumbling teeth cannot be cured by Homeopathy.** They require filling, extraction of teeth and dentures which need a qualified dentist. Lesser problems and pains in teeth and gums can be managed with Homeopathy.

**Decay of Teeth**

Some common symptoms and medicines which are to be taken two times a day are given below:

- **With loss of enamel. Pain if food touches teeth.** Calc flour 200.
- **With pain from cold or hot food. Teeth sensitive.** Carbo Veg 200. Sensodyne toothpaste may be used.
- **Teeth dark and crumbling.** This is common with those who smoke and usually affect teeth in upper jaw. Kreosotum 30. **Carbo Veg and Kreosotum are incompatible.**

**Grinding of Teeth**

Some common symptoms and medicines which are to be taken two times a day are given below:

- **Grinding by day with pain.** Belladonna 200.
- **Grinding at night or in sleep.** Podophyllum 200

**Pyorrhoea**

Pyorrhoea is a problem of the gum. **There is discharge of pus, loosening of teeth and bad breath.** Symptoms and medicines to be taken two times a day are:

- **With bleeding and retracted gums.** Carbo Veg 200.
- **When pus and foul smell is predominant.** Merc Sol 200 and Silicea 200

**Toothache**

In case of toothache without any associated symptoms give alternate doses of Hekla Lava 30 and Merc Sol 200 every 4 hours till the pain is gone. In other cases, given below, take the suggested medicine three times a day:

- **Toothache in tooth with cavity.** Antim Crud 200.
- **Toothache caused by air current or anything hot or cold.** Calcarea Carb 30 alternate with Carbo Veg 200.
- **Toothache worse after warm drink or extraction.** Arnica 200 and Chammomilla 200.
- **Toothache along with pain in left eye and face.** Spigelia 200.

**Laryngitis**

**Laryngitis causes hoarseness and at times temporary loss of voice. See a throat specialist if problem persists.** Some common symptoms and medicines which are to be taken two times a day are given below:

- **On exposure to dry cold air. Fever present.** Aconite 30
- **With suffocating cough. Throat red. Swallowing difficult.** Belladonna 200.
- **With severe pain and smelly sputum.** Carbo Veg 200.
- **With hoarse cough, worse at night, after drinking and laughing.** Drosera 200 and Phosphorous 200.

- **With scanty sputum. There is great hoarseness with barking cough. Severe pain from ear to ear when swallowing or turning head. Worse in the morning.** Hepar Sulph 200.

**Pharyngitis**

**Pharyngitis is an inflammation of the throat. There is fever with chill and headache.** Some common symptoms and medicines which are to be taken two times a day are given below:

- **Throat painful and burning. Uvula, a small fleshy portion hanging at the back of the throat swollen. Swallowing painful. Severe pain in post nasal region running into ears.** Merc Cor 30.
- **Pain from ear to ear. Swelling of throat. Ulcers with pus. Constant desire to swallow.** Merc Sol 200.

# 10

# Problems of Heart and Lungs

## Heart or the Circulatory System

It is not possible for a layman to diagnose heart problems. Serious heart problems are best treated by experienced doctors, be they Allopathic, Homeopathic or Ayurvedic. However, once a diagnosis has been made and the patient decides to have Homeopathic treatment because he cannot afford Allopathic treatment, options are available. Some of them are discussed in the succeeding paragraphs.

### Arterial Thrombosis

Arterial Thrombosis is the formation of a blood clot in an artery of the brain, heart or leg. There is a sudden pain in the affected part. A clot in the brain leads to a stroke and has been discussed under the Chapter on First Aid. Start treatment with Bothrops 30 which is supposed to dissolve the clot. Dissolve 10 pills in half a cup of water and administer one tea spoon of the medicine every half hour. Additional medicines are:

- **Pain and stirring of the clot on the inner side of leg or thigh.** Apis 1000 two times a day.
- **Pain in the artery of the heart. The skin of the area is swollen, blue and cold.** Continue Bothrops 30, one dose two times a day after the dissolved medicine is finished.
- **Pain in an artery while the patient is asleep. Worse left side.** Lachesis 200, two times a day.

### Arterio- Sclerosis

**Arterio-Sclerosis is the disease in which the walls of the arteries get hardened and narrowed due to fatty (cholesterol) deposits. This causes**

**high blood pressure, chest pain or pain in left arm from elbow to shoulder, dizziness and pain or cramps in legs after exercise.** If there is weakness and the person tires easily, it could be a serious problem. One or more arteries may be blocked and surgery may be required. Seeing a doctor and getting a proper test done is a must. ECG will only show a problem if it is serious.

As an interim measure take 6 pills of Arnica 200 and Crataegus 30 two times a day till pain ends. Continue with Crataegus 200, once a day for a month.

**Blood Pressure – High**

**Blood pressure 140/80 is normal, 160/90 is high and 170/95 is dangerously high. High blood pressure can lead to a stroke or heart attack. It must be kept below high level. The first medicine is Veratrum Virde 30 which should be taken two times a day till blood pressure falls below 140/90.** A blood pressure measuring machine should be available at home for those who can afford and use it. Additional medicines based on symptom which should also be taken two times a day are:

- **A feeling that the heart stops beating for a few seconds; with violent headache, double vision and sleeplessness.** Aurum Met 200 and Gelsemium 200.
- **With weakness, dizziness, breathlessness and palpitation.** Glonoine 200

**Blood Pressure – Low**

**Blood pressure should be considered low if it falls below 90/60. It is an indication of a weak heart and can lead to heart failure.** One must see a doctor.

Caffeine 200 should be taken two times a day till the blood pressure reaches 100/60 Other medicines based on symptoms which should also be taken two times a day for a month are:

- **With pain in region of the heart.** Cactus 30.
- **With weak digestion, lack of appetite and acidity.** Carbo Veg 200.
- **Chronic low blood pressure.** Crataegus Q, 10 drops in water four times a day. Must see a specialist as early as possible.

**Chest Pain**

Chest pain or pain in the region of the heart and often extending to the arm or shoulder can be of different types:

- **Coronary Thrombosis or Heart Attack. The pain is very severe.** Please see Heart Attack in Chapter 7 on First Aid.
- **Angina Pectoris or pain in heart. The pain usually comes on account of fatigue and is not very severe. Increase in frequency of attacks and severity of pain are dangerous signs of an impending heart attack and a heart specialist should be consulted.** If you decide to treat with Homeopathy, start with one dose of Arnica 1000. Thereafter, take 6 pills of Arnica 200, Crataegus 200 and Gelsemium 200 till pain disappears. Continue for three days thereafter.
- **Chest pain or heart attack due to mental shock.** Arnica 1000 and Tabacum 30 two times a day for a week or till patient stabilizes.
- **At times chest pain is attributed to heart burn on account of gas due to indigestion. This wrong assessment cost Grandpa's father-in-law his life. Never take a chance. Always treat chest pain as a heart problem and treat it as given above. It will cause no harm.**

**Palpitation**

**Palpitation is a disagreeable awareness of heart beat. The patient can hear his own heartbeat. Patient should see a doctor if problem persists.** Some common symptoms and medicines which are to be taken two times a day for a week are given below:

- **Palpitation with anxiety, fainting and tingling in fingers. Pain in chest or left shoulder.** Aconite 30, Arnica 200 and Phosphorus 200.
- **Palpitation. Heart seems to stop beating for two to three seconds.** Arnica 200 and Aurum Met 30.
- **Violent palpitation from least exertion.** Belladonna 200 and Spigelia 200.
- **Palpitation with irregular pulse rate. In women at approach of menstruation. With vertigo, breathlessness and flatulence.** Arnica 200 and Cactus 30.
- **Palpitation with breathlessness while climbing a mountain.** Coca 30 and Glonoine 200.
- **Least movement causes palpitation. Weak pulse.** Digitalis 30.
- **Palpitation with rapid pulse rate.** Veratrum Alb 200.

**Rapid Pulse Rate**

A pulse rate above 90 should be considered excessive pulse rate. The patient should lie down and rest. Administer Arnica 200 and Cactus 30 two times a day for a week.

**Slow Pulse Rate**

**A pulse rate below 60 is considered slow pulse rate. One must see a doctor.** Administer Digitalis 30 and Carbo Veg 200 two times a day till pulse rate rises above 70.

**Bronchial Asthma**

The patient has periodic attacks of wheezing, breathing difficulty and coughing. First aid for an attack has been explained in the Chapter on First Aid. **Bronchial Asthma is better treated with allopathic medicines and one should see a doctor. Nebulizers gave great relief to Grandma when she had Asthma attacks.**

Some common symptoms and medicines which are to be taken two times a day along with allopathic medicines are given below:

- **Attacks come at night or after midnight.** Arsenic Alb 200.
- **Asthma with chronic cold.** Bacillinum 200.
- **Sudden attack. It seems the patient would suffocate.** Belladonna 200.
- **With great breathing difficulty. Chest painful to touch.** Calcarea Carb 200.
- **Attack during wet cold weather.** Dulcamara 200.

**Colds and Coughs**

Some common symptoms and medicines which are to be taken two times a day are given below:

- **Coughing with white sputum which is difficult to take out and loud rattling sound during breathing.** Antim Tart 200.
- **Dry cough with little or no sputum. Pain in chest.** Bryonia 200.
- **Cold with breathing difficulty, breathing difficulty and wheezing.** Ipecac 200.
- **Cold with sticky yellow/green sputum.** Kali Bi 200.
- **Cold with thick yellow/green slimy sputum and cough.** Pulsatilla 30.
- **Violent cough with thick, yellow and lumpy sputum.** Silicia 200.
- **Violent cough leading to vomiting.** Ipecac 200.

If you find it too confusing take some off the counter cough syrup. Drinking hot pepper Rasam or soup can do wonders. If the patient feels feverish and has body pain, it is flu and for medicines see under fevers.

**Pneumonia**

**Pneumonia is a dangerous disease and can lead to fatality. There is high fever, persistent cough, rapid breathing and pain in the chest. Sputum may sometimes contain blood. The patient should be taken to the hospital at the earliest.** In the interim, start treatment by dissolving 10 pills of Aconite 30 in half a cup of water and administer one spoon every 30 minutes. Once this is finished give Aconite 200 and Carbo Veg 200 two times a day till the patient is all right. If there is excessive blood in sputum, also give Ferrum Phos 30 two times a day along with the other medicines. If symptoms do not improve in two days give Arsenic Iod 30 in place of Aconite 200. If possible, see a doctor as early as possible but keep administering Aconite 200 and Carb Veg 200 till the patient is admitted into a hospital.

**Snoring**

Administer Opium 200, two times a day for a month.

**Tuberculosis**

**Tuberculosis can be of any part of the body but tuberculosis of the chest is most common. There is severe weakness, persistent coughing with blood in sputum and pain in the chest. Free treatment is usually available at all government hospitals.** In Homeopathic treatment, start with Bacilliam 200, two times a day for three days. There after give Allium Satvium 30 and Arsenic Iod 30, two times a day for at least a month.

**Weakness of Lungs**

**The patient loses elasticity or capacity of the lungs. There is difficulty in breathing and blowing. There is enlargement of the chest but loss of weight.** Some common symptoms and medicines which are to be taken two times a day for a week are given below:

- **Coughs and coughs. Pain in chest. Breathing difficult.** Ammonium Carb 30 and Carbo Veg 200. Carbo Veg should be continued for a month or more.
- **Total breathlessness.** Arsenic Alb 200 and Carbo Veg 200. Carbo Veg should be continued for a month or more.

# 11

# Problems of the Digestive System

**Appendicitis**

**Appendicitis is an inflammation of the appendix, a small part in the right side of the lower abdomen. There is severe pain.** Initially it may come and go. Later the pain becomes continuous and unbearable. Pain is worse on movement. There is also nausea, vomiting and foul breath. **The disease is life threatening and immediate surgery is recommended to remove the appendix. The patient should be given 6 pills of Belladonna 200 and 6 pills of Silicia 200 and taken to the hospital.** If surgical facility is not available, continue the medicines for times a day till the patient improves. If available give 4 pills of Belladonna 1000 instead of Belladonna 200. Once pain subsides continue the medicine for three days. The give 10 pills of Lycopodium 200 or 4 pills of Lycopodium 1000 for seven days to stop recurrence.

**Stomach Pain**

Stomach pain could be due to various reasons. **If pain is severe, take whatever painkiller you have in the house and try to get to a hospital or doctor.** Some symptoms and medicines to be taken three times a day are given below:

- **Pain radiating from the navel.** Argentum Nit 200.
- **Sudden severe pain. Belladonna** 200.
- **In the region of the liver or right side.** Berberis Vulgaris 200 and Chelidonium 30.
- **Pain on left side of the stomach.** Ceanothus 30.

- **Pain with convulsions** Cicuta 200
- **Pain traveling from right side of stomach to left.** Lycopodium 200.

**Cholera**

Cholera is a dangerous, infectious, disease usually caused by contaminated water or food. It assumes epidemic form after floods and other natural disasters. The patient has profuse diarrhoea, vomiting, cramps and dehydration. **The patient must be evacuated to a hospital as early as possible.** But that may not be possible during epidemics after floods or natural disasters. The patient must be given complete rest and plenty of fluids in the form of oral re-hydration agents or water with sugar or glucose and a pinch of salt. Some symptoms and common medicines are:

- **Dry cholera with scanty stool and vomiting.** Camphor 200.
- **With copious rice water like stool and constant vomiting.** One dose of 10 pills of Verat Alb 1000 to start with. Repeat after six hours if required. If Veratrum 1000 is not available, give Verat Alb 200, 10 pills, three times a day.
- **In case of cholera with cramps in abdomen and calves give** Cuprum Met 200, three times a day in addition to Verat Alb 200 or 1000.
- **In case of blood and gas in stool,** give Carbo Veg 200 in addition to Verat Alb 200 or 1000.

**Eructation**

Eructation means ejecting gas in the stomach noisily through the mouth. Some symptoms and medicines to be taken two times a day are given below:

- **Foul smelling and tasting of food recently taken.** Antim Crud 200.
- **Sour tasting with heaviness of stomach.** Carbo Veg 200.
- **After eating lots of green vegetables or fatty food.** Bitter taste. Pulsatilla 30.

**Flatulence or Gas**

Excessive formation of gas in the stomach or intestines is a common problem in many persons. There is a feeling of heaviness. Some symptoms and medicines to be taken two times a day are given below:

- **Gas pressure upwards and downwards. Eructation and flatulence both with relief from both. No appetite.** Carbo Veg 200
- **Gas pressure upwards and downwards. Hungry at meal times. No relief from eructation or passing flatus. Better from movement.** China 200.
- **Pressure downwards. Stomach is bloated. Rumbling in intestines. Constipation could be present. Worse after meals.** Aloe 200 and Lycopodium 200.

**Gall Stones**

Gall stones are stone like solids formed in the gall bladder (located in the liver). These can be detected by Ultra Sound techniques. The problem is quite common. **Silent gall stones (gall stones which do not cause pain) are not treated in Allopathy. Painful stones are removed by surgery.** Painless gallstones should be treated with Chelidonium 30 and Calcarea Carb 200, two times a day for at least a month and then one dose a week. **Painful gallstones should be removed by surgery within 48 hours**. In the interim treat with Berberis Vulgaris 200, China 200 and Chelidonium 30 two times a day for a week or till pain disappears. Chelidonium 30 should be continued for at least a month. There are also a number of readymade Homeopathic combinations for gallstones.

**Hepatitis or Jaundice**

Jaundice is usually caused by water borne infection from drinking contaminated water or eating roadside contaminated food. Skin, eyes and tongue turns yellow. There is bitter taste in the mouth. **It is a life-threatening disease. Doctors do not treat the disease but the causes.** Viral Hepatitis gets cured on its own as the liver begins to heal. If it is due to a blocked bile duct, surgery may be necessary. However, that can only be detected after a scan. The patient should be given complete rest. **The patient should be given mainly boiled foods. All fats and oils should be completely removed from the diet. The patient should be given plenty of sugar cane juice, fruit juices and glucose water. Alcoholic drinks are prohibited during jaundice.** Give Chelidonium 30 and Chionanthus 30, two times a day for at least a month.

Some home remedies of jaundice are as under:

- Mix quarter teaspoon of turmeric powder in a cup of hot water and drink it 2 to 3 times a day.

- Make a paste of tender papaya leaves and take it with one teaspoon of honey.
- Put 8 to 10 leaves of lemon in one cup of boiling water. Cover, keep for five minutes and then drink the water.

**Liver Abscess**

The symptoms are pain in the region of the liver (on the right side of stomach just below the ribs) when walking, coughing or touching the region. **It is a serious disease and one should see a doctor if pain persists.** Give Siliceca 200 three times a day till the pain disappears completely.

**Liver Enlarged**

When liver is enlarged and painful to touch and there is itching of skin or anaemia. **See an allopathic doctor.** In the interim or in parallel give two doses of Merc Sol 200 per day till pain disappears.

**Stomach Upset**

Stomach upset could lead to loose motions, acidity, vomiting and flatulence. Some symptoms and medicines to be taken two times a day till cured are given below:

- **From over eating or eating too much of fatty food. Tongue is white and there is loss of appetite.** Antim Crud 200.
- **With pain in region of navel. Vomiting and belching. Mild stomach upset.** Argentum Nit 200.
- **Violent stomach upset with loose motion. Vomiting and pain may be there. Possible food poisoning.** Veratrum Alb 200 and Arsenic Alb 200.
- **When nausea and vomiting are the most important symptoms.** Ipecac 200 and Arsenic Alb 200.
- **In patients with irregular eating habits or after a night of heavy drinking and eating.** Nux Vomica 200.
- **If mucus seen in stool.** Merc Sol 200 and Arsenic Alb 200.

# 12

# Problems of the Urinary System

**Bloody or Cloudy Urine**

**When colour of urine is red or cloudy; the patient's face is swollen; there could be severe headache and backache; urine is passed in large quantities and the patient is always thirsty; the problem is serious and a doctor should be consulted as early as possible.** Some symptoms and medicines to be taken two times a day are given below:

- **Burning sensation and pain while passing urine.** Cantharis 200 and Terebinthina 30.
- **Turbid brown urine. High blood pressure.** Phosphorus 200 and Terebinthina 30.
- **When accompanied by watery diarrhoea.** Phosphorus 200 and Arsenic Alb 200.

**Burning**

**Sometimes there is a burning sensation while passing urine. The urine may be passed drop by drop. Sometimes the discomfort persists for some time after the urine is passed.** Administer 6 pills of Sulphur 200 and Cantharis 200 alternately two times a day till cured.

**Diabetes**

Diabetes is a disease where the body does not produce enough insulin to use the sugar intake. The excess sugar accumulates in the blood and urine and leads to many other medical problems like heart attack, delay in healing of wounds, gangrene or rotting of flesh in the body due to lack of blood circulation and eye problems like cataract. Blood sugar test is the most reliable way of finding out whether one is diabetic or not. Those who are obese and have sedentary habits or a family history of diabetes are most likely to be affected by the disease. The early symptoms are abnormal thirst, increase in frequency of urine both during day and nights and ants frequenting the place where urine has been passed. The patient tires easily. There is numbness of hands and feet and ulcers develop on the feet.

**Diabetes cannot be cured but can be controlled through strict control of diet and medication.** The patient must stop taking sugar, sweets, butter and reduce intake of fried food. The patient must also take brisk walk for half an hour at least five times a week.

Syzygium Jambobalanum reduces the sugar in blood and urine. Deciding the dosage is the difficult part. **Sudden drop in sugar level in blood can lead to extreme lethargy, sweating and collapse. Diabetic patients should always carry some toffees on them and take these if they feel lethargy and discomfort.**

The patient should be given 10 drops of Syzygium Jambolanum mother tincture three times a day before meals to start with. The number of drops can be increased or decreased based on blood tests. If the PP sugar level is over 300, give 15 drops, three times a day. Where testing facilities are not available, the dose has to be adjusted based on the comfort level of the patient. **Do not give Homeopathic or Ayurveda drugs for diabetes if the patient is already on Allopathic medicines. It may cause drastic drop in blood sugar and lead to collapse and even death.**

Some additional medicines which are to be taken three times a day based on symptoms are given below till the symptoms disappear:

- **On presence of ulcers on feet.** Acetic Acid 30.
- **Pain and bruised feeling in muscles. Presence of boils.** Acid Phosphoric 200.
- **Extreme thirst. No appetite. Signs of gangrene i.e. appearance of black patches on skin.** Arsenic Alb 200
- **Rheumatic pain in joints. Good appetite.** Lactic Acid 200.

**Inability to Control**

Some Symptoms and medicines to be taken two times a day are:

- **Small quantity passes involuntarily with burning.** Apis Mel 200.

- **Passes involuntarily day and night.** Argentum Nitricum 200
- **Sudden intolerable urging.** Cantharis 200 and Thuja 200.

**Inability to pass Urine**

Some symptoms and medicines to be taken two times a day are given below:

- **Due to no apparent reason.** Aconite 30.
- **With stinging pain.** Apis 200.
- **Due to Urinary infection.** Belladonna 200.
- **Due to fright.** Opium 200.
- **Cannot urinate without passing stool.** Apis 200

**Kidney Stones**

**Kidney stones are difficult to detect without ultrasound investigation. The common symptoms are severe pain in lower back on one or both sides of the backbone reaching down to lower abdomen and groin.** The problem is serious and one should consult a doctor as early as possible. Berberis Vulgaris 30 and Urtica Urens 30 taken three times a day can expel the stones without surgery. There are also some Homeopathic combinations like Dr. Reckwegs' R 27 – Renocalcin which are also effective in removing kidney stones without surgery.

**Smelly Urine**

Some symptoms and medicines to be taken three times a day are given below:

- **Repulsive odour. Brown colour.** Benzoic acid 30.
- **Smells of ammonia. Horse urine.** Nitric Acid 200.

# 13

# Problems Related to Rectum and Stool

**Constipation**

**Constipation is difficulty in passing of tools. It is a fairly common problem. Unless treated, it can lead to other problems of the anus like piles and fissures.** The most important part of the treatment is to include lots of fibrous food like brown bread, oats, wheat porridge, vegetables and fruits in the diet. Taking "Isabgol" and drinking two to three glasses of water as soon as one gets up in the morning will help. Start treatment with 10 pills of Sulphur dissolved in half a cup of water and sipped on an empty stomach. No other medicine that day. Some symptoms and medicines to be taken two times a day are given below:

- **No desire. Total inability to pass stool. Stool dry, hard and knotty.** Bryonia 200 and Alumina 30.
- **No desire for days. Gas. Stool initially hard but later liquid and gushing.** Antim Crud 200 and Lycopodium 200.
- **Desire but no ability. Stool large and difficult to expel. Anus torn and bleeding.** Nat Mur 200.
- **No desire for days. No discomfort. Stool hard dark balls.** Opium 200.
- **Desire but difficulty in passing stool. Face becomes red while straining to pass stool. Piles.** Causticum 200.
- **No desire, no stool for days. Piles and fissures which burn and itch. Obese persons.** Graphites 200.

**Piles**

**Piles are a problem of swollen veins inside and outside the anus.** There is frequent bleeding while passing stool or even otherwise. There can be pain or itching. The primary medicine is Nitric Acid 200 which should be taken three times a day. Additional medicines to be taken two times a day along with Nitric Acid based on specific symptoms are:

- **Veins protruding like grapes. Intense itching and burning. Involuntary passing of stool.** Aloe 200.
- **With oozing mucus. Undergarments get soiled.** Antim Crud 200.
- **Violently painful. Burning. Sensitive to touch.** Belladonna 200.
- **Where there is profuse bleeding.** Hamamelis 200.
- **In patients with liver problems and gas.** Lycopodium 200.
- **When pain and burning are the main symptoms.** Ratanhia 30

**Diarrhoea**

**Diarrhoea is passing copious watery stool. There is risk of the patient getting dehydrated which in turn can cause fatality.** The patient should be given "Oral Re-hydration" medicine or six to eight glasses of a solution of glucose or sugar and a pinch of salt every day. Some symptoms with medicines to be taken two times a day are as under;

- **Profuse watery stool:** Phosphorous 200 and Veratrum Alb 200.
- **Stool is green, fetid, and profuse. Worse early morning.** Podophyllum 200 and Veratrum Alb 200.
- **Copious watery stool passes involuntarily.** Apis Mel 200 and Veratrum Alb 200.

**Dysentery**

**Dysentery is due to infection of the intestines.** The patient frequently passes large quantities of watery stool. There is risk of the patient getting dehydrated which in turn can cause fatality. The patient should be given "Oral Re-hydration" medicine or six to eight glasses of a solution of glucose or sugar and a pinch of salt every day. Some symptoms and medicines to be taken three times a day are given below:

- **Amoebic Dysentery. Frequent passing of watery stool with cramps in the abdomen.** Administer Emetine 200 and Ipecac 200 alternately.

- **Blood Dysentery.** Administer Merc Cor 30 and Hamamelis 200 alternately.
- **Mucous Dysentery. Slimy stool with jelly like mucous.** Alternate Merc Sol 200 and Aloe 200.
- **Blood and Mucous.** Sulphur 200 if Merc Sol fails.
- **Dysentery with pain in thighs extending into the legs.** Rhus Tox 200.

**Food Poisoning**

**Food poisoning is caused by taking spoilt or contaminated food. The contamination may be due to small animals or insects like rats or cockroaches or flies falling into the food while it is being cooked. The patient has stomach pain, vomiting and diarrhoea.** The Arsenic Alb 200 and Argentum Nit 200 should be administered three times a day. If there is continuous rice water coloured thin diarrhoea, give one does of Veratrum Alb 1000 once a day till diarrhoea stops. Give the patient "Oral Re-hydration Solution (ORS)" or water mixed with sugar and a pinch of salt and plenty of fluids like sugar cane or fruit juices to stop dehydration.

**Involuntary**

Some symptoms and medicines to be taken twice a day are:

- **Involuntary passing of solid large ball of stool.** Aloe 200
- **Involuntarily during excitement or during sleep.** Hyoscyamus 200.
- **Involuntary passing of large quantity of liquid stool.** Phosphorus 200 and Secale 30.

**Urge to Pass Stool**

**Sometimes there is a sudden urge to pass stool. The person just cannot wait and has to rush to the toilet.** Some symptoms and medicines which are to be taken two times a day for a week are given below:

- **There is sense of insecurity as to whether gas or stool will pass. Stool passes without effort almost unnoticed.** Aloe 200
- **Great urge early in the morning.** Podophyllum 200 and Lilium Tigrinum 30.
- **Rumbling and rolling of gas in stomach. Watery stool and gas gushing out.** Croton Tig 30.
- **Diarrhoea painful, watery, copious, forcefully evacuated at night.** Veratrum Alb 200.

# 14

# Problems Related to Back and Locomotor System

**Back Pain**

Some symptoms and medicines to be taken two times a day for a week or more are given below:

- **Lower back and hips ache just above tail bone. No strength in legs. Worse from standing, stooping, walking or motion.** Aesculus 30
- **Violent back pain from waist to tail bone. Sensation of heavy weight on tailbone.** Antim Tart 200.
- **Pain to back, spine or neck due to injury or strain. Can be old injury.** Arnica 200 / 1000 and Hypericum 200.
- **Pain in lower back in the region of the kidneys. Worse lying down.** Berberis Vulgaris 200 and Calcarea Carb 200.
- **Pain in the small of the back with stiffness caused by exposure to cold wet weather or strain. Better from motion and lying on hard surface.** Rhus Tox 200.
- **Pain in back with stiffness, particularly in the small of the back. Better with pressure and worse from movement.** Bryonia 200.
- **Backache early morning before rising due to flatus which could not escape.** Staphysagria 200.

**Neck Pain**

Some symptoms and medicines to be taken two times a day for a week or more are given below:

- **Painful and stiff neck. Head drawn to the left.** Chelidonium 30.
- **Spasms and cramps in the muscles of the neck.** Cicuta 200.
- **Cervical spondylosis.** Cimicifuga 200. Take along with allopathic medicines and Analgesics.

**Tail Bone Pain**

Some symptoms and medicines to be taken two times a day for a week or more are given below:

- **Pain at base of spine caused by a shock or jolt.** Ruta 200 and Conium 200.
- **Severe pain in tail bone due to injury.** Arnica 1000 and Hypericum 200.

- **Severe pain in tail bone. Must sit still.** Worse getting up from sitting position. Lachesis 200.

**Ankles**

Some symptoms and medicines to be taken two times a day are given below:

- **Severe pain in ankles and in the bones of the feet.** Ammonium Carb 30.
- **Ankles swollen, legs weak and trembling.** Argentum Met 30.
- **Sprain due to injury. Start treatment with one dose of Arnica 1000. Then administer** Bryonia 200 and Ruta 200, two times a day.

**Blue Hands and Fingers**

Hands and fingers of some young women are cold and blue due to poor blood circulation. Some common symptoms and medicines which are to be taken two times a day are given below:

- **Cold blue skin.** Arsenic Alb 200 and Carbo Veg 200.
- **Cold blue nails.** Nitric Acid 200.

**Corns and Callosities**

Corns and callosities can form on palms, fingers, toes and feet due to prolonged pressure among sportsmen and ordinary people due to ill-fitting hoes. Corn caps are available over the counter and can be used for removing them. Some even cut the hard portions with shaving blades. **Corn caps**

**must never be used by persons with diabetes. Nor should diabetic persons ever cut the hard portions of corns.** This can lead to diabetic gangrene. Grandpa's friend had to have his leg amputated after a barber cut his corn and the wound turned septic and developed gangrene. **One simple way of softening hard corns is to soak some cotton in apple cider vinegar and cover the corn overnight with the help of bandage or sticking plaster.** Some symptoms and medicines to be taken two times a day are given below:

- **Large inflamed painful corns.** Antim Crud 200.
- **Callosities on soles of the feet. Toes and fingers contracted.** Lycopodium 200.
- **Corns caused by ill-fitting shoes.** Sulphur 200.
- **Corns or and callosities of sportsmen.** These should be softened by method explained above. Arnica 200 and Antin Crud 200.

Thuja mother tincture should be applied on the corns for relief.

**Feet**

Some problems with symptoms and suggested medicine to be taken two times a day are given below:

- **Feet cold, damp and sweaty.** Calcarea Carb 30.
- **Burning of soles.** Sulphur 200
- **Burning and itching of feet and soles.** Calcarea Sulph 30.
- **Pain and stiffness in bones of feet.** Phytolacca 200 and Ruta 200.

**Hands**

Some problems with symptoms and suggested medicine to be taken two times a day are given below:

- **Pain in hand. Hard nodes form on the joints.** Actea Spicata 30 and Ledum 200.
- **Icy coldness and numbness. With or without pain.** Aconite 30.
- **Involuntary shaking of hands.** Mag Phos 200 and Agaricus 200.

**Heels**

Some problems with symptoms and medicines to be taken two times a day are given below:

- **Severe pain in heel and feet due to growth of heel bone.** Aranea Diadema 30 and Calcarea Flour 1000.
- **Pain in heel as from treading on a pebble.** Lycopodium 200.
- **Severe pain, as if pinched by too narrow a shoe, particularly at night.** Chelidonium 30.

**Hips**

Some problems with symptoms and suggested medicine to be taken two times a day are given below:

- **Severe pain in hip, worse left side.** Aesculus 30 and Colocynthis 200.
- **Severe pain in hip, worse right side.** Aesculus 30 and Chelidonium 30.
- **Hip and thigh feel lame, especially after lying down.** Aconite 200.
- Hip joint stiff. Movement difficult. Calcarea Flour 30 and Petroleum 30.

**Knees**

Some problems with symptoms and suggested medicine to be taken two times a day are given below:

- **Chronic rheumatic inflation of knee joints. Very painful. Walking and sitting on the floor difficult.** Ledum 200, Calcarea Flour 30 and Sticta 30.
- **Sharp pain in knees, ankles, calves and soles.** Canibis Indica 30. **If swelling is there also take** Apis 200.
- **Left knee painful.** Colocynthis 200.
- **Right knee painful.** Jacaranda 30.
- **Crackling sound while moving all joints, especially knee.** Angusta Vera 30 and Causticum 200.
- **Knee stiff. Cannot bend.** Petroleum 30.
- **Pain in the knee in diabetic patients.** Lactic Acid 30 and Sticta 30.

**Legs and Calves**

Some problems with symptoms and suggested medicine to be taken two times a day are given below:

- **Legs and feet cold. Swelling present.** Colchium 30.
- **Painful stiffness in calves. Sudden loss in strength. Difficult gait.** Conium 200.
- **Swelling of feet and legs. Legs and feet sweat at night.** Merc Sol 200.

- **Pain in legs, ankles, feet, heels, toes and underside of thighs. Worse in the morning.** Phytolacca 30.
- **Pain in bones.** Eupator Perf 200.

**Loss of Coordination of Muscles**

**This results from diseases of the brain or spinal cord.** The movement of the patient is clumsy. He finds it difficult to keep his balance. Some common symptoms and medicines which are to be taken two times a day are given below:

- **Jerking, twitching and trembling of hands and feet accompanied by itching. Palsy of upper and lower limbs due to weakness of spinal cord.** Mag Phos 200 and Agaricus 200.
- **Staggering gait. Walks stooping forward.** Manganum Aceticum 30 and Conium 200.
- **Constant or involuntary nodding of head.** Aurum Sulph 30.
- **Retarded child. Legs and hands weak and trembling. Twitching of whole body.** Bufo 30.
- **Due to epileptic attacks.** Hyoscyamus 200.
- **Cannot walk on uneven ground.** Lilium Tig 30.

**Myasthenia Gravis**

It is a rare chronic condition where the muscles all over the body tire with very little exertion. Eyelids may droop. This is a serious condition and one must see a doctor. **Homeopathic medicines which can be tried are Causticum 1000, six pills once a week to be taken for three to six months.**

**Nails**

Some common symptoms and medicines which are to be taken two times a day are given below:

- **Toe nails brittle.** Antim Crud 200
- **Crippled nails with white spots.** Silicea 200.
- **Brittle or crumbling nails.** Thuja 200
- **Pain in Finger nails.** Berberis Vulgaris 200.
- **Painful and pus-filled nails.** Silicea 200

**Numbness of Hands and Fingers**

Some common symptoms and medicines which are to be taken two times a day are given below:

- **Numbness and tingling due to exposure to cold air or due to shock, grief or fear.** Aconite 30.
- **Numbness of hands and fingers after sleep or in the morning.** Lachesis 200.

**Paralysis**

Paralysis is inability to move our limbs in the normal fashion, particularly hands or legs. Some symptoms and medicines to be taken two times a day are given below:

- **Gradually appearing paralysis of legs, hands, eyelids, face etc.** Aconite 200 and Causticum 200.
- **Right sided paralysis.** Causticum 200 and Crotalus 200.
- **Left sided paralysis.** Lachesis 200.

**Shoulders**

Some problems with symptoms and suggested medicine to be taken two times a day are given below:

- **Constant pain under right shoulder bone.** Chelidonium 30.
- **Pain in right shoulder.** Sticta 30 and Phytolacca 30.
- **Pain in left shoulder.** Asparagus 30 and Onosmodium 30.
- **Frozen shoulder.** Cannot lift the arm or take it behind ones back. Lactic Acid 30. Physiotherapy if accessible should be taken.

**Strains**

Some problems with symptoms and suggested medicine to be taken two times a day are given below:

- **Strain affecting muscles.** Arnica 200, Bryonia 200 and Rhus Tox 200.
- **Strain affecting tendons.** Arnica 200 and Ruta G 200.

**Thighs**

Some common symptoms and medicines which are to be taken two times a day are given below:

- **Contraction of hamstring muscles.** Ammonium Mur 200.
- **Pain in thigh muscles which comes in spasms.** Plumbum Met 30
- **Intense shifting pain in thighs and legs.** Pulsatilla 30
- **Tearing pain in thighs with or without dysentery.** Rhus Tox 200.

**Toes**

Some common symptoms and medicines which are to be taken two times a day are given below:

- **Eczema of toes or fingers with or without loss of nails.** Borax 200.
- **Painful swelling of toes, ankles or fingers.** Actea Spicata 30.
- **Painful swelling of great toe.** Ledum 200 and Benzoic Acid 30.

**Itching between Toes is common in athletes whose feet remain wet due to perspiration inside shoes or people who work in water for long periods like rice farmers. There is severe itching between toes. The skin becomes pulpy and comes off.** The treatment should start with one dose of Sulphur 200 and be followed with two doses of Bacillium 200 every day.

**Varicose Veins**

**Varicose veins are swollen and twisted veins seen on the surface of thighs and legs.** There is a dull pain after standing for some time. There can be leg cramps at night. It is caused by increased blood pressure in the veins of the legs due to inadequate blood circulation and standing for long periods. **Varicose veins can also indicate weakened or damaged heart valve and this should be investigated by ECG.** Three simple ways to treat varicose veins before they get very bad are; exercising to improve blood circulation of the legs as per advice of a physiotherapist; wearing compression stockings and keeping feet raised while resting with the help of pillows or cushions. One should reduce salt intake to reduce water retention and increase intake of potassium. (Refer Chapter 1)

If treated with Homeopathy, one dose of Sulphur 200 should be given to start treatment in all cases. Some common symptoms and medicines which are to be taken two times a day are given below:

- **Best medicine as a preventive and cure.** Pulsatilla 30.
- **Chronic cases in old persons or women who have borne many children.** Pulsatila 30 and Calcarea Flour 200.

**Whitlow**

**Whitlow is a painful infection in the skin next to the finger nails of the hand.** Some common symptoms and medicines which are to be taken two times a day are given below:

- **Severe pain. The nail loosens and comes off.** Hepar Sulph 200.
- **When caused by puncture by a needle.** Ledum 200.
- **In old cases where there is pus formation.** Silicea 200.

**Wrist & Arm**

Some common symptoms and medicines which are to be taken three times a day are given below:

- **Cramps in fore arm with weakness and trembling.** Gelsemium 200.
- **Pain in bones of arms or wrist.** Eupator Perf 200
- **Painful stiffness in wrist and right arm.** Phytolacca 30.
- **Pain or pain of wrist, arm and fingers due to over use.** Ruta 200.

**Cramps**

**A cramp is a sudden seizure in a limb with severe pain. It can be due to exhaustion and dehydration or otherwise.** It is a fairly common problem. Taking "Oral Re-hydration Slats (ORS)" helps prevent cramps due to loss of body fluids. Some symptoms and medicines to be taken two times a day are given below:

- **Cramps in calves, sole or palms.** Cuprum Met 200 and Calcarea Carb 200.
- **Cramps in feet, calves, hands etc with pain like electric flashes.** Cuprum Met 200 and Veratrum Alb 200.
- **Cramps in hands and fingers.** Anacardium 200 and Ambra Gresia 30.
- **Cramps in writers, typists, sitarists, pianists, violinists, sportsmen etc due to excessive strain.** Ruta 200 and Mag Phos 200.

**Pain in Heel**

Some common symptoms and medicines which are to be taken three times a day are given below:

- **Due to growth of heel bone.** Calcarea Flour 1000 and Aranea Diadema 30.
- **Pain in heel as though treading on a pebble.** Lycopodium 200.

# 15

# Problems of Skin

**Barbers Itch**

**This is a rash which affects the faces of men.** Some common symptoms and medicines which are to be taken two times a day are given below:

- **Moist eczema or itching pimples around the mouth or on the chin.** Graphite 200.
- **Oozing eczema with pus in hair follicles.** Sulphur Iod 200.
- **The rash is red, swollen and there is intense itching.** Rhus Tox 200.

**Bed Sores**

**Bed-ridden patients develop bed sores around elbows and buttocks. It first appears as a red patch on the affected part. If not treated immediately, the skin cracks, gets infected and forms a sore.** Arnica 200, taken three times a day as a preventive as soon as redness is seen. Calendula Q mother tincture should be externally applied to the sore area. **Treatment should be started with one dose of Sulphur 200,** which should be repeated every four days. **When multiple boils are formed or there are dark red itching blotches.** Sulphuric Acid 200.

**Blisters**

**When a clear fluid accumulates under the skin due to heat or friction or any other reason, it is called a blister. Never burst or puncture the blister as it may get infected.** Some common symptoms and medicines which are to be taken two times a day are given below:

- **A blister caused by insect bite.** Apis 200 or 1000.

- **When caused due to burn or friction (common in sports persons playing racquet games).** Cantharis 200. Also apply Cantharis mother tincture externally three to four times a day.
- **When infected with pus and shooting pain.** Silicea 200.

**Boils or Abscess**

**An Abscess or boil is formed when pus is formed due to infection. There is swelling and severe pain. A carbuncle is a collection of boils.** Some common symptoms and medicines which are to be taken two times a day are given below:

- **Abscess deep in the muscles in neck or thighs.** Silicea 200 and Calcarea Carb 30.
- **Abscess with hard edges.** Silicea 200 and Calcarea Flour 30.
- **If Silicea fails to cure try** Myristica 200.
- **Carbuncles with stinging pains, burning and swelling.** Apis 200 and Anthracinum 30.
- **Boils with offensive discharge.** Arsenic Alb 200 and Silicea 200.
- **Carbuncles or ulceration near anus or genitals.** Thuja 200.

**Bruises**

**A bruise is the discoloration of the skin due to an injury sustained in an accident or fight. The skin usually turns purple or blue. There is pain and swelling. Apply ice pack but do not massage.** Give Arnica 200 two times a day internally and apply Calendula mother tincture or ointment externally.

**Burns**

Take Cantharis 200 internally and apply Cantharis mother tincture (ten drops in half a tea cup of water) or Cantharis ointment externally. Also see under Chapter on "First Aid." It is desirable to see a doctor if pain persists or blisters appear. **Immediate hospitalization is a must in serious cases.**

**Cracks in Skin**

Some common symptoms and medicines which are to be taken three times a day are given below:

- **Cracks around the mouth, in nipples, at the end of fingers, between toes or around anus.** Graphites 200.
- **Painful cracks on hands and feet.** Hepar Sulph 200.

- **Cracks in hands, feet and lips which occur during winter.** Petroleum 200.

**Eczema**

**Eczema is a troublesome skin problem which takes time to cure.** First there is redness which is followed by swelling, itching, formation of blisters and sometimes oozing of fluid. The blisters ultimately dry and form scabs and crusts. **One can try to abort eczema by making a fresh emulsion of one teaspoon of mustard oil and one teaspoon of water and apply it to the red area twice a day.**

Some symptoms and medicines to be taken two times a day are given below:

- **Dry eczema.** Arsenic Alb 200.
- **Moist and oozing eczema.** Graphite 200.
- **On eyelids.** Graphite 200 and Bacillium 200.
- **On anus.** Graphite 200 and Berberis Vulgaris 200.
- **On palm of hands.** Anacardium 200 and Selenium 200.
- **On scrotum and genitals.** Graphite 200, Cantharis 200 and Rhus Tox 200. Also apply Cantharis mother tincture after diluting it with five times the quantity of water.
- **On forehead and cheeks which are painful to touch.** Graphite 200 and Ledum 200.
- **On the head or behind the ears.** Take Calcarea Carb 200 and Lycopodium 200.

**Expulsion of foreign Bodies**

**Sometimes foreign bodies like fish bones, thorns, wood splinters or broken sewing or injection needles get lodges in body tissues and are difficult to remove.** Give Silicea 200 two times a day till discomfort disappears.

**Gangrene**

**Gangrene is death of tissues of the body due to infection caused by injury followed by rotting of the flesh. The most commonly affected parts are fingers, legs and toes. It happens due to inadequate blood circulation in the affected parts.** The skin of the area first turns pale and then black and spreads. Severe pain may or may not be felt at the periphery of the affected area. It is a serious problem. **If neglected, the part may have to be**

**amputated to save the person's life.** Some symptoms and medicines to be taken two times a day are given below:

- **Gangrene in diabetic persons.** Arsenic Alb 1000, Silicia 200 and Carbo Veg 200.
- **Gangrene in bed ridden or inactive persons starting in the toes.** Silicia 200 and Carbo Veg 200.
- **Dry gangrene in old people with shrivelled skin.** Carbo Veg 200 and Secale 30.

**Herpes**

**Herpes is a skin problem which appears as a tiny pus-filled blister on red skin. The area may soon be covered with a cluster of such blister which is very painful. The patient may have fever. Herpes can affect any part of the body. If possible, it is better to go to an allopathic doctor for quick relief.** Some symptoms and medicines to be taken two times a day are given below:

- **Except on genitals.** Hepar Sulph 200 and Rhus Tox 200.
- **On genitals.** Hepar Sulph 200 and Nitric Acid 200.
- **If the blisters are bluish and very painful and itchy.** Hepar Sulph 200 and Ranunculus Bulbosus 30.

**Itching**

Itching or desire to scratch an affected area is a common problem. It can be due to various reasons. The treatment should be started with one dose of Sulphur 200 and to be repeated once a day. Some common symptoms and medicines which are to be taken two times a day are given below:

- **Severe allergic itching on any part of the body.** Aconite 30 or 200.
- **Severe itching in folds of skin in thighs or behind knees.** Aethusa 30 and Causticum 200.
- **Ring worm or itchy rash on the head.** Dulcamara 200.
- **Severe itching accompanied by swelling.** Hepar Sulph 200.
- **Small pimples all over the body which itch violently.** Mag Sulph 30. Also apply Mag Sulph mother tincture externally or Mag Sulf 30 in liquid form, 3 to 4 times a day.

- **Severe itching in orifices like eye lids, lips, urethra, anus or in persons with unclean habits who do not bathe. Itching which is aggravated by washing or is worse at night.** Sulphur 200.

**Leukoderma**

**Persons affected by Leukoderma suffer from formation of white patches on the skin due to de-pigmentation. The disease is neither infectious nor contagious. There is no pain or loss of sensation.** The treatment should start with one dose of Tuberculinum 200 which should be repeated once a month. Also administer Hydrocotyle 30, two doses a day for three to four months. The affected part should be exposed to sunlight for about 15 minutes, once a day, half an hour after administering the medicine.

**Lice**

**Lice are small parasites that live in the hair on the skin and suck blood. Lice spread from one person to another by contact.** Some common symptoms and medicines which are to be taken two times a day are given below:

- **Lice in hair on the head.** Carbolic Acid 30.
- **Lice in hair on the body.** Lycopodium 200.
- **Lice in pubic hair.** Staphysagria 200.

**Numbness**

**Numbness is loss of sensation in a part of the body. It may be a sign of leprosy. A doctor must be consulted if the problem is not cured by Homeopathic medicines within a week.** Some common symptoms and medicines which are to be taken two times a day are given below:

- **Numbness caused by fear, anguish, sudden financial loss or exposure to cold air.** Aconite 30.
- **Numbness with tingling in lips, tongue, knees, legs or feet.** Nat Mur 200.
- **In collapse due to cholera.** Veratrum Alb 200 or 1000.

**Odour**

Some common symptoms and medicines which are to be taken two times a day are given below:

- **Offensive body odour.** Hepar Sulph 200.
- **Offensive odour in pus, perspiration, saliva, urine, stool, mouth or ear.** Merc Sol 200.

**Perspiration / Sweating**

Some common symptoms and medicines which are to be taken two times a day are given below:

- **Cold sweat due to illness or excessive sweating of the head which wets the pillow.** Calcarea Carb 30.
- **Non-stop sweating. Sour sweat.** Hepar Sulph 200.
- **Excessive sweating. Sweat has foul odour.** Merc Sol 200.
- **Excessive sweating in skin folds like armpits, leg pits.** Sulphur 200.

**Pimples**

**Pimples are a very common problem particularly with young women and children. Proper diet is an important part of the cure.** Avoid fats, chocolates and dry fruits. Take plenty of fresh fruits and vegetables and drink plenty of water. Start treatment with one dose of Sulphur 200 and repeat once a week. Some common symptoms and medicines which are to be taken two times a day are given below:

- **In adolescence.** Asterias Rubens 30.
- **Pus filled pimples** Merc Sol 200.
- **Pus filled and painful.** Hepar Sulph 200.

**Prickly Heat**

**Prickly heat is skin rashes which develop on the body in summer heat.** They feel scratchy. Apply Syzygium Jambobalam mother tincture on the affected area. Some common symptoms and medicines which are to be taken two times a day are given below:

- **In folds of skins around neck, armpits or chest.** Causticum 200.
- **Red with intense itching.** Rhus Tox 200.

**Ring Worm**

**Ring worm is a skin fungus that is highly contagious. It starts as a small red itchy patch on the skin and grows into a ring that keeps growing larger.**

One can try to abort the infection by making a fresh emulsion of one spoon of mustard oil and one spoon of water and applying it on the red patch twice a day. Bacillium 200 and Sepia 200 are the basic medicines and should be taken two times a day alternately. Also take Apis 200 or 1000 if there is swelling, burning and intense itching.

**Warts**

**Warts are small growths on the skin.** Some common symptoms and medicines which are to be taken two times a day are given below:

- **Hard, painful warts on hands.** Antim Crud 200.
- **Warts on eye lids, eye brows, face.** Causticum 200.
- **Moist oozing and painful warts.** Nitric Acid 200.
- **Warts like raisins (fig warts)** Thuja 200 or 1000. Also apply Thuja mother tincture.
- **Fig warts with severe itching and burning.** Sabina 30. Also apply Sabina mother tincture.

# 16

# Women's Medical Problems

**Anaemia**

**Anaemia is a common blood disease among women. The number of red cells in the blood is less than what is necessary for the body to function properly. It is mostly due to malnutrition, iron deficiency, Vitamin B12 deficiency and heavy menstruation. The patient tires easily and feels dizzy.** In some cases, the patient suffers from head ache, shortness of breath, palpitation and lack of sleep. Diet containing natural iron like raw banana, spinach (Palak), apples, roasted potatoes etc help preventing anaemia. A vitamin C tablet a day improves absorption of iron from natural sources. **Amla (Goose berry) is rich in both iron and Vitamin C. It can be taken raw, in juice form or as a sweet pickle (Murabba).** In cases of severe anaemia or on conceiving, the woman should consult a doctor and get medicine or tonic.

Some symptoms and Homeopathic medicines to be taken two times a day are given below:

- **Great weakness with pain in the head.** Ferrum Phos 30 and Iridium 30.
- **After childbirth.** Acetic Acid 30 and Iridium 30.
- **Due to menstrual irregularities.** Nat Mur 200 and Iridium 30.
- **After malaria or other disease.** Arsenic Alb 200 and Iridium 30.

**Breast Abscess**

The affected area of the breast is red and painful. The patient may have fever. Administer Phytolacca 30 and Silicea 200 two times a day. Apply Phytolacca mother tincture externally to soothe the inflation. **Also get examined for breast cancer if over 40 years.**

**Hard knots in Breast**

Administer Calcarea Flour 200 two times a day for four weeks. Increase potency to Calcarea flour 200 after two weeks and continue for another two weeks. **If the patient is above 40 years, get check done for malignancy.**

**Breasts Underdeveloped**

**Some women are genetically pre-disposed to having small breasts. In some, post puberty under-developed breasts may be due to medical reasons.** The woman may like to see a doctor to check. The Homeopathic medicines for under developed breast to be taken two times a day for two to three months are as under:

- **Underdeveloped breasts in young women.** Sabal Serrulata 3x or 30
- **Breasts lax and shrunken, hard and painful to touch.** Nipples also painful. Conium Mac 30.

**Nipples**

Some symptoms and medicines to be taken two times a day are given below:

- **Nipples inflamed. Tender to touch. Very painful.** Chamomilla 200.
- **Nipples painful. Want to press breasts hard to get relief.** Conium 200
- **Cracked, painful and tender nipples.** Graphites 200 and Nitric Acid 200.
- **Nipples drawn in and sore.** Silicea 200.

**Pain in Breasts**

Some symptoms and medicines for painful breasts to be taken two times a day are given below:

- **Pain in breast during menstruation time.** Bryonia 200.
- **Breasts become larger and painful before menstruation.** Conium 200.
- **Pain in breast, particularly left breast.** Asterias Rubens 30.

**Leucorrhoea**

**Moderate quantity of odourless, colourless discharge from female genital organs is normal. It is not a problem and can be present during pregnancy. But excessive, coloured or smelly discharge needs to be treated.** Eating boiled Lady's Finger or two ripe bananas per day may reduce the problem.

Some symptoms and medicines to be taken two times a day are given below:

- **Foul smelling white discharge with burning sensation.** Argentum Met 200 and Hepar Sulph 200.
- **Milky white.** Calcarea Carb 200.
- **Brown discharge.** Lilium Tig 200.
- **Thick, profuse as menstrual blood with pain in small of back and thighs.** Mag Sulph 30.
- **Thick, yellow or greenish with pain. Vagina feels raw.** Pulsatilla 30
- **During first few weeks after childbirth.** Rhus Tox 200.
- **Very painful. Discharge as thick as curd. Offensive smell.** Sepia 200.
- **Copious burning discharge with pain in genitals. Burning sensation in Vagina. Vulva itching.** Sulphur 200.

**Menstruation – Absence (Amenorrhea)**

**Menstruation stops when women become pregnant, when breast feeding or at menopause. Menstruation may stop due to other reasons too like excessive exercise, mental stress, too less or too much body fat.**

Some symptoms and Homeopathic medicines to be taken two times a day are given below. If in doubt take two medicines which are closest to your problem.

- **On account of great weakness and anaemia.** Ferrum Met 30.
- **Absence of menstruation with digestion problems, palpitation or abdominal cramps.** Kali Carb 200.
- **When accompanied by severe headache and leucorrhoea.** Sepia 200.
- **When stopped by fright**. Opium 200
- **On reaching age of puberty. Breasts do not develop.** Pulsatilla 30 and Lycopodium 200.

**Menstruation - Irregular**

**There are many causes of irregular menstruation.** It could be due to stress and other lifestyle factors like excessive exercise and inadequate calorie intake, birth-control pills, uterine polyps or fibroids, hormone imbalance, thyroid being too high or too low, cysts on ovary etc. **It is best to see a gynaecologist and gets adequate tests done to eliminate the presence of serious medical problems.** Some home remedies for irregular periods include doing yoga, maintaining a healthy bodyweight, increase intake ginger (one can chew chopped raw ginger with a little salt in the morning), increase intake of cinnamon, ensure adequate intake of vitamin B6, D and calcium.

Some symptoms and Homeopathic medicines to be taken two times a day are given below. **If in doubt take two medicines which are closest to your problem.**

- **Irregularity of time and quantity.** Nux Moschata 30.
- **Starts, stops and starts again. There could be clots of blood.** Pulsatilla 200 and Coccus Cacti 30.
- **Too frequent, profuse with clotted blood.** Ammonium Carb 30.

**Menstruation – Profuse (Menorrhagia)**

**The symptoms of Menorrhagia are soaking up more than one sanitary napkin or tampon per hour, need to wake up and change sanitary protection at night, bleeding for a week or longer, passing large blood clots, having to stop normal activity due to bleeding and getting symptoms of anaemia like excessive tiredness. One must see a doctor if these symptoms are there and if there is inter period bleeding or any vaginal bleeding after menopause.** Some common causes of Menorrhagia are hormone imbalance, improper functioning of ovaries, uterine fibroids or polyps, use of IUD and even uterine cancer.

Some symptoms and Homeopathic medicines to be taken two times a day are given below. If in doubt take two medicines which are closest to your problem.

- **Too early. Profuse. Blood bluish. Worse at night.** Ambra Grisea 30.
- **Too early, profuse and painful.** Arsenic Alb 200
- **Too early, profuse and painful. Pain comes and goes suddenly. Discharge is blood red and foul smelling.** Belladonna 200 and China 200.
- **Too early, profuse, lasts a long time. Some times with vertigo and toothache.** Calcarea Carb 200.
- **Non-stop menstruation. One period runs into the next. Great weakness.** Carbo Veg 200 and Nux Vomica 200.
- **Early, profuse, large clots of dark blood while passing Urine.** Coccus Cacti 30.

- **Haemorrhage from uterus, clots with long strings, blood dark, black, slimy.** Crocus 30.

**Menstruation - Painful**

Some symptoms and medicines to be taken two times a day are given below. If in doubt take two medicines which are closest to your problem.

- **Pain like labour pain. Comes and goes. Short duration.** Belladonna 200 and Chamomilla 200.
- **Pain with abdominal and pelvic soreness. Worse on movement.** Bryonia 200.
- **Pain across pelvis, hip to hip.** Cimicifuga 200.
- **Pain just before flow starts. Menstruation with cramps.** Mag Phos 200.
- **Pain in vagina, pelvic region and back.** Sepia 200.
- **Pain during menstruation with great weakness.** Veratrum Alb 200.
- **Haemorrhage during climacterics with palpitation and flashes of heat.** Lachesis 200.

**Menstruation – Scanty (Hypomenorrhea)**

Scanty menstruation or short periods usually occur at puberty or when approaching menopause. This is not a serious problem. However, **scanty periods in 20s and 30s could be due to thyroid dysfunction, polycystic ovary syndrome or perimenopause. In such cases you should see a doctor and have a check-up.**

Some symptoms and Homeopathic medicines to be taken two times a day are given below. If in doubt take two medicines which are closest to your problem.

- **Early, short duration, scanty with great weakness. Followed by transparent, burning leucorrhoea.** Alumina 200.
- **Scanty menstruation with severe headache.** Bryonia 200.
- **Painful and extremely scanty menstruation. Lasts less than a day.** Euphrasia 200.
- **Scanty, irregular or late and painful. Starts, stops, flows and stops. Blood dark, thick and clotted.** Pulsatilla 30 and Lilium Tig 200.
- **Scanty menstruation with pain in small of the back.** Sepia 200.
- **Menses very late, scanty, for short duration. Blood thick and black. Vagina and vulva sore. Worse on washing.** Sulphur 200.

### Menopause

**The cessation of the menstrual cycle occurs in women sometime in mid-forties. This is a problematic stage for women. They suffer from both psychological and physical problems. There could be depression.** The woman also feels flushes of heat.

Some symptoms and Homeopathic medicines to be taken two times a day are given below. If in doubt take two medicines which are closest to your problem.

- **Flushes with convulsions. Worse in the sun, working in the kitchen or stooping.** Glonoine 200.
- **Palpitation, breathlessness, weakness, headache and bleeding uterine. The patient may have piles or suffer from high blood pressure and depression.** Lachesis 200 and Sanguinaria 30.
- **Flushes of heat, perspiration and weakness. There is a sensation that the uterus is coming down. Vagina painful on coitus. Severe headache.** Sepia 200
- **Excessive bleeding at the time of menopause. Also, burning and smelly leukorrhea.** Argentum Met 30.
- **Mental depression and Irritability.** Ignatia 200 and Lachesis 200.
- **Pain in uterus. From hip to hip.** Cimicifuga 200 and Sepia 200.
- **Palpitation during menopause. Headache and flushes of heat.** Lachesis 200.

### Ovarian Cyst

**Formation of cysts in the ovary may not show any symptoms. Pain may be experienced in the lower abdomen during menstruation. Pain may also be experienced during coitus, while passing stool, frequent need to urinate and irregular periods.** It is not a serious problem. However, **if there is bleeding from the ovary outside periods, pelvic pain with fever, nausea and vomiting, one must see a doctor.**

Some symptoms and Homeopathic medicines to be taken two times a day are given below:

- **Severe pain in lower abdomen. The patient draws up double or pulls her knees up to the chest.** Colocynthis 200.
- **Vagina dry. Coitus painful.** Lycopodium 200.

**Pregnancy Related Problems: Abortion**

Most abortions are spontaneous. The foetus is expelled before the 20th week of pregnancy. The most common symptom is vaginal bleeding. There may be pains at regular intervals like labour pains. **If a pregnant woman is involved in an accident or fall, immediately administer a dose of Arnica 1000 to reduce chances of abortion.** The woman must be made to lie down at the first hint of vaginal bleeding or discharge of water and given maximum rest. **A doctor should be consulted as early as possible.** Some symptoms and medicines to be taken two times a day are given below:

- **Tendency to miscarriage.** Give Sabina 30 till the end of the third month.
- **If haemorrhage starts.** Crocus 30
- **In case of fear and anxiety during pregnancy.** Aconite 30.

**Debility and other Problems**

**Many women suffer from great weakness during pregnancy. Most of the cases are due to inadequate nutrition and rest.** Some symptoms and medicines to be taken two times a day are given below:

- **Backache during pregnancy.** Aesculus 30.
- **Physically run-down condition. Weakness.** Carbo Veg 200.
- **Anaemia with or without headache.** Ferrum Phos 30.
- Mentally run-down condition due hard work. Excessive albumin in urine. Helonias 30 and Carbo Veg 200.
- **Veins enlarged. Varicose veins during pregnancy.** Hamamelis 200.
- **Excessive albumin in urine. Nausea in pregnancy.** Merc Cor 30.

**Morning Sickness**

**Morning sickness consists of nausea, vomiting and sometimes heart burn. It usually begins five to six weeks after conception and continues till the sixteenth week. The primary medicine is Ipecac 200 which should be administered twice a day for a few weeks.** Some symptoms and additional medicines to be taken two times a day are given below:

- **Nausea and vomiting in the morning while eating or immediately after eating or drinking. Violent hiccups.** Nux Vomica 200.
- **If vomit is of milky mucus.** Sepia 200.
- **Excessive vomiting with great weakness.** Arsenic Alb 200.

- **With bitter eructation or eructation with smell of food taken. Great desire for taking sour things.** Pulasatilla 30.

**Milk Problems**

Mother's milk is the best food for an infant. However, there can be problems during lactation. Some symptoms and medicines to be taken three times a day are given below:

- **If there is failure of secretion of milk, give Agnus 30 for a month.**
- **If milk is deficient give Asafoetida 30 a day for a month.**
- **If milk bloody.** Bufo 30.
- **If milk sour, rejected by child. Anaemia during nursing.** Acetic Acid 30
- **If milk salty, rejected by child.** Calcarea Phos 30.
- **Milk too profuse.** Lac Caninum 30. Helps dry up milk.
- **Nipple very sore during nursing.** Croton Tig 30.

**Post Natal Care**

A woman requires great care after childbirth. She must get adequate nourishment and rest. One dose of Kali Carb 200 and Carbo Veg 200 per day helps the patient to regain her strength.

**Polyps and Warts**

Polyps are small soft growths on the skin of any organ like the nose or vagina. Warts on the other hand are small, hard, abnormal growths on the skin. Some symptoms and medicines to be taken three times a day are given below:

- **Uterine polyps. There may be slight bleeding from the urethra.** Phosphorous 200.
- **Warts on the vagina, vulva or lower abdomen.** Thuja 1000. Apply Thuja mother tincture.

**Uterus Problems: Bearing Down**

**When the ligaments holding the uterus, the bladder and the rectum become weak, the uterus shifts out of its position. There is a bearing down sensation as though everything will escape through the vagina. At times there is a physical protrusion of the uterus through the vagina.** One must see a doctoe.

Some symptoms and medicines to be taken two times a day are given below:

- **Constant, violent bearing down sensation. Relieved by standing. Worse lying down.** Belladonna 200.
- **Pelvic pain rising towards the breasts.** Murex 30.
- **Strong bearing down sensation. Uterus has to be stopped physically from coming out. Worse standing.** Sepia 200.

**Tumour in Uterus/ Ovaries**

Benign tumours in the uterus are common in women above 35 years. They are difficult to detect, particularly in the initial stages. The patient may suffer from excessive and painful menstruation. It is always advisable to see a doctor and have a proper check-up if there is pain in uterus or ovary.

Some symptoms and medicines to be taken two times a day are given below:

- **Tired feeling in limbs. Limbs become numb easily. Hot burning feet. At times shivering all over.** Kali Iod 200.
- **Enlargement of uterus with chronic inflammation.** Aurum Mur 30
- **Ovarian tumour.** Apis 200.

**Urinary Infection**

**It is a common disorder with women.** The infection can come from the bladder or the vagina. Urine is passed more frequently than at normal times. Passing urine is painful. There is burning sensation while passing urine. To ease the problem, take lots of water. Urinate as often as required. It helps to flush the infection out. One should take probiotics or good bacteria. Take Vitamin C tablets. Wipe from front to back. Practise good sexual hygiene like urinating before and after sex, using condoms and washing genital before and after sex. One may take one dose of Cantharis 200 as a preventive after using public toilets.

Some symptoms and medicines to be taken two times a day are given below:

- **Burning in urethra with pain and burning.** Aconite 30. Start treatment with this medicine.

- **Great urging with cutting pain before, during and after passing urine. Urine is very hot.** Cantharis 200.
- **Urethra sore. Sudden desire to urinate which cannot be controlled. Painful coitus.** Thuja 200.

**Conclusion**

**Women tend to be shy and do not like to discuss their medical problems with male members including their husbands. They mostly suffer in silence.** They must get over this shyness and discuss their problems with other older ladies. **When in doubt, consult a doctor**

Women in the house should be made to read this chapter. In case they are unable to read and understand English, it should be read and explained to them by an educated woman. Homeopathic medication can relieve pain and discomfort in most cases. **However, if there is no improvement in three to seven days, they must see a doctor and get treated.**

# 17

# Sexual Problems of Men and Women

**Sex is no longer a taboo, either among men or women.** Education about sex starts in school. On line pornography is easily accessible on mobile phones. Contraceptives of various kinds are available over the counter. Abortion is legal in most parts of the world. Live in arrangements have replaced marriage even in some third world countries like India. Thus, competition has entered the bedroom. Performance in the bedroom has a major effect on relationships. **If one has any problems, it is best to see a competent doctor and get treated. The treatments given in this chapter are for the bashful or the timid. They may or may not work. Treatment takes a few weeks to months to show results. Do not expect an instant solution like a Viagra tablet.**

Grandpa also feels that masturbation is good both for men and women. It provides a solution when one is hot but there is no partner or the partner is unwilling. It reduces stress, marital rape and sexual assault against minors. In men over 60, it may prevent prostrate problems.

## Male Sexual Problems

### Strong Desire

Some symptoms with suggested medicines to be taken two times a day are.

- **Strong desire.** Erection is painful. Cantharis 200
- **High and uncontrollable sexual excitement.** Tarentula Hispanica 30.
- **Prolonged morning erections.** Pulsatila 30

**Hydrocele or Swollen Balls**

This problem results from accumulation of fluid. Some symptoms and medicines to be taken two times a day are given below:

- **Testicles swollen but hard and painless.** Merc Sol 200 and Calcarea flour 200.
- **Testicles swollen, hard and painful.** Aurum Met 30.
- **Testicles extremely painful with fever.** Rododendron 30.
- **Testicles swollen but soft and painless.** Silecea 200.
- **Testicles swollen, retracted and very sensitive to touch.** Pulsatilla 30.

**Impotence**

**Impotence is the inability of the male to have sexual intercourse due to inability to have or maintain an erection. It is mainly a psychological problem.** Some times this could be a temporary problem caused by excessive sexual activity. It will go away in a week's time.

If it a persistent problem, six pills Argentum Nit 200 should be taken an hour or two before going to bed. This is to reduce anxiety that the person will not be able to get and maintain an erection.

Some symptoms and medicines to be taken two times a day are given below:

- **Low sexual vitality. No desire. No erection.** Agnus 30.
- **Deficient erection.** Lycopodium 1000. 6 pills to be take once a week only.
- **Strong desire but weak erection.** Sulphur 200. A combination of Sulphur 200, Calcarea Carb 200 and Lycopodium 200 taken twice a day in that order is the best for weak erection. Continue for a week or two till problem is gone.
- **Loss of desire. Weak erection. Premature discharge.** Sulphur 200, Phosphorous 200 and Omosmodium 200.

**Pain**

Some symptoms with suggested medicines to be taken twice a day are as under;

- **Pain in spermatic cord, testicles and prepuce.** Berberis Vulgaris 200.
- **Prolonged painful erection.** Camphor 30.

**Premature Ejaculation**

**In this case ejaculation takes please too soon before the woman reaches her orgasm.** Six pills of Argentum Nit 200 should be taken one to two hours before going to bed to reduce anxiety about ability to satisfy partner. Some symptoms and medicines to be taken two times a day are given below:

- **Discharge too quick.** Calcarea Carb 200 and Bufo 30.
- **Discharge without erection.** Gelsemium 200.
- **Discharge on mere contact of bodies.** Sulphur 200.

**Prostate Problems**

The prostate gland is found only in men and produces seminal fluid. It is located at the base of the penis beneath the bladder and in front of the rectum. **There are two types of prostrate problems, enlargement (hypertrophy) and inflammation (prostatism).** Enlargement of the prostate gland in men cause difficulty in passing urine. The patient takes a long time to urinate. **If the patient urinates more than two or three times at night, if there is urge but there is delay in starting to urinate, if urination is painful and accompanied by low back pain and fever, it could be a case of prostate cancer and one must see a specialist at the earliest.The patient must eliminate or reduce smoking, alcohol, spicy food, junk food, chlorinated drinks, tomatoes and tomato products.**

Some symptoms with suggested medicines to be taken two times a day are as under:

- **Dribbling and numbness in penis after passing of urine.** Baryta Carb 200
- Excessive itching and irritation of the urine passage for the entire length of the penis. **There is no force and the person cannot urinate without standing with feet wide apart and leaning forward.** Chimaphila 30
- **Prostate enlarged. Intermittent urination in old people. See Chapter on Problems of the Aged.**
- **Partial paralysis of bladder. Almost unable to urinate.** Gelsemium 200.

**Testicles Retracted**

Some symptoms and medicines to be taken three times a day are given below:

- **Testicles retracted, painful, worse right side.** Clematis 30
- **Testicles retracted, swollen and painful. Worse left side.** Rododendron 30.
- **Testicles retracted, swollen and very sensitive to touch.** Pulsatilla 30.

## Female Sexual Problems

### Frigidity

Frigidity is aversion of women to sex. It may be due to various reasons like excessively conservative family background, sexually abused or molested as a child or even being a lesbian. **It is best to see a psychologist to understand the problem.**

Some symptoms and medicines to be taken two times a day are given below:

- **Definite aversion to coitus in timid women.** Graphites 200.
- **Aversion to coitus in emotional and moody women.** Ignatia 200.
- **Desire diminished.** Berberis Vulgaris 200.
- **Sexual desire completely destroyed.** Onosmodium 200.

### Nymphomania

Some women suffer from an insatiable and uncontrolled desire for sex play and coitus. **The first medicine to be given three times a day is Pulsatilla 30.** Some symptoms and additional medicines to be taken three times a day are given below:

- **With urinary problems like excessive urging and pain.** Cantharis 200.
- **In hysterical women. Early and copious menstruation and titillation in vulva and vagina.** Moschus 30.
- **Lively, nervous and affectionate women. Least touch of sexual parts causes violent sexual excitement.** Murex 30.
- **Severe itching in vulva. Erotic spasms during menstruation.** Tarentula Hispanica 200.

### Painful Coitus

Some symptoms with suggested medicines to be taken two times a day are as under:

- **Constriction of vagina due to physical weakness and tiredness. The patient wants to be left alone.** Gelsemium 200.
- **Vagina dry and constricted. Constipation is present.** Lycopodium 200.

# 18

# Life Style Diseases

## Obesity

Obesity is putting on excess weight. It comes from eating more than what is used by the body, the excess being converted to fat. **There are five main reasons for obesity, thyroid problem, poor eating habits consisting of too much carbohydrates, fats and fast food, constant snacking and lack of exercise.** The first thing that the patient needs to do is to get Thyroid test done and get treated if it is not all right. If Thyroid test is negative then obesity is due to over eating and lack of exercise.

**Many people suffer from eating disorders or excessive snacking.** They usually have some domestic problem which makes them unhappy. They compensate their unhappiness by the pleasure of eating and slowly they get addicted to snacking like getting addicted to alcohol or tobacco. They then keep eating between meals, in mid-morning, in the afternoon or even in the middle of the night. They take care to hide their snacking habits from other family members. **Controlling obesity with medicines is just not possible unless one can control ones eating and exercise. Psychological treatment to overcome eating disorder may be necessary before obesity can be tackled.**

Some symptoms and medicines to be taken two times a day for a month is given below:

- **Patient suffers from suppressed anger, anxiety and depression. Desires for company. Tired lower extremities. Worse from slightest exertion.** Calcarea Ars 200. Women may also take Ignatia 200.
- **Patient is fat, fair, and flabby and perspires a lot.** Calcarea Carb 200.
- **Thyroid enlarged. Obstinate constipation.** Fucus Vesiculosus 30.

- **The patient is irritable, restless, head strong and flies into a rage over trifles. Often suffers from frontal headache, weak but rapid pulse.** Thyroidinum 30
- **The obese person has heart problems and rheumatic pains.** Esculentine Q. Take onetablespoon in half cup of warm water twice a day.

Phytolacca Berry mother tincture or pills can be taken with the above medicines. Walking for half an hour is a must. There are also some Homeopathic combinations. Medication can be continued for more than a month if improvement is seen. **However, please remember, nothing will work if you are eating too much carbohydrate and fast food and burning less calories than what you are eating.**

**Migraine**

**Migraine is a severe recurring headache. It can be accompanied by nausea and vomiting. The Patient can often predict its coming.** Some symptoms and suggested medicines, to be taken two to three times a day are given below. There are also some homeopathic combinations which are quite effective:

- **Due to mental exertion. Pain better on tight bandaging and pressure. Pain in bones of the head.** Argentum Nitricum 200.
- **Violent throbbing headache, throbbing temples, hot flushed face, better from pressure, worse from light, noise, jolts, lying down and in the afternoon.** Belladonna 200.
- **Attack preceded by excitement and talkativeness.** Cannabis Indica 30.
- **Due to acidity and liver problems.** Chionanthus 30.
- **With severe pain in eye sockets. During journey.** Cocculus 200.
- **Due to grief or anger, especially women. Feels as if nails being driven into the head from the sides.** Ignatia 200.
- **On waking up after sleep. Pain at root of the nose. Pressure and burning on vertex. Due to exposure to sun. Vision becomes dim.** Lachesis 200.
- **During hangover. Feels if a nail is being driven into the top of the head.** Nux Vom 200.
- **Due to over work. Pain starts in the right temple and wanders through the head.** Pulsatilla 30.
- **Pain on left side and during menses.** Sepia 200

**Liver Cirrhosis**

**Cirrhosis of the liver is its gradual degradation which comes from excessive drinking. It leads to liver failure and death.** The problem is difficult to diagnose because there are no major symptoms or pain. The indications of possible cirrhosis are loss of appetite with tiredness and weakness, disinterest in sex and a feeling of numbness in the extremities. **It is a serious problem and needs specialist medical attention.** In the interim or in parallel give Chelidonium 30 and Nux Vomica 200 two times a day for at least a month. Drinking addicts should be given 10 pills of Chelidonium 30 and Nux Vomica 200 once a week as a preventive.

**Fatty Liver Disease**

It is a common lifestyle disease. **Excess fat gets stored in the liver and can lead to liver damage.** The signs of fatty liver disease can be abdominal swelling, enlarged spleen, red palms and jaundice. The condition can be caused by obesity, diabetes or high triglycerides. It can also be caused by excessive drinking. Persons suffering from fatty liver problem should avoid full fat cheese, full cream yoghurt, red meat, foods fried in palm or coconut oil and sugary items like candy. **Fatty liver problem in persons who drink heavily can be cured by stopping drinking for two weeks. In others, a change in eating habits will help. Fatty liver could also be a side effect of taking corticosteroids, anti-depressants and anti-psychotic medications and tamoxifen. Coffee is good for non-alcoholic fatty liver.**

**Homeopathic medicines** for fatty liver disease are Chelidonium 30 and Phosphorus 200, twice a day for two weeks.

**Severe and Persistent Stomach Ache (Dyspepsia)**

**Dyspepsia is a pain or severe discomfort felt in the upper and middle region of the stomach. The pain sometimes comes and goes. It may remain for a long time. One may feel too full while eating and stop. One may not feel hungry at all. The pain is most severe immediately after a meal. It is a life style disease and can affect people of all ages.** The disease could be due to stress, lack of adequate sleep and exercise, missing breakfast and irregular eating habits.

The symptoms may be an indication of a serious disease like stomach ulcer or even cancer. **If pain is severe and persistent, one must see a doctor and get a thorough check-up done.**

To cure dyspepsia naturally, one must avoid too much fried food, chocolates, onions and garlic; take water instead of aerated drinks, reduce or stop intake of coffee and alcohol. One should eat small meals but eat more times; control one's weight and not were tight clothes. Over the counter anti acids may cure it in early stages.

**Homeopathic medicines for Dyspepsia are Abies Nigra 200 and Nux Vomica 200** to be taken twice a day for a week and then one doe every week.

**Constipation**

**Constipation means difficulty in passing stool.** The main causes could be life style (not eating enough fibre in the form of vegetables, not drinking enough water, not getting enough exercise, irregular habits including meal timings and going to sleep. Eating large amounts of cheese, mental stress and deliberate attempt to delay bowel movements for reasons like travelling, shopping, attending classes or meetings etc. can also cause constipation). The other reasons could be side effects of medicines, medical conditions or pregnancy. **One must see a doctor if there is pain, presence of blood in stool and "irritable bowel syndrome".**

Natural way of treating cancer include drinking more water, adding fibre to your diet by taking more vegetables and fruits, exercise more, drink coffee, take **herbal laxatives like "Isabgol". Taking probiotic food like yogurt, tempeh, pickles, butter-milk and supplements also help.** There are a number of Ayurvedic formulations for constipation but Grandpa has not tried out any.

Homeopathic medicines to be taken two times a day are as under:

- **Obstinate constipation, no urging for days. Stool hard. Rectum full.** Alumen 200 and Bryonia 200.
- **Large stool. Has to strain before and during motion. Face turns red while straining.** Alumina 30 and Causticum 200.
- **Constipation with flatulence. First stool hard and then soft.** Lycopodium 200.
- **Frequent desire. Each time only a small amount passes.** Nux Vom 200.

**Piles or Haemorrhoids**

Piles or haemorrhoids are swollen veins in one's anus. They can be inside the rectum (blind piles) or around the anus. **Primary reason for piles is chronic constipation.** The other possible reasons could be regular heavy lifting, pregnancy, obesity and having anal intercourse. **One must see a doctor if there is bleeding, change in bowel habits and stool changes colour and consistency.** The best way to prevent piles is to keep stool soft. The home remedies are the same as for constipation given above. In some cases, like pregnancy, piles may get all right by itself. In early stages one can apply over the counter ointments and go for home remedies. Neglected, painful, bleeding piles may require surgery.

Some symptoms and Homeopathic medicines are as under:

- **Protruding like grapes. There is itching, burning and insecurity of rectum.** Aloe 200.
- **With continuous oozing of mucus. Underwear gets soiled.** Antim Crud 200.
- **Haemorrhoids protrude while urinating.** Berberis Vulgaris 200.
- **Haemorrhoids red, intensely painful, swollen and sensitive to touch. In persons with liver problems and flatulence.** Lycopodium 200.
- **If there is bleeding add Hammamelis 200.** Apply Hammamelis mother tincture on the anus.
- **Blind or Internal piles which are painful, and secrete blood and pus.** Nitric Acid 200 and Nux Vom 200.

**Neck Pain**

Neck pain can be caused by poor posture, repetitive movements, sleeping with the neck in awkward positions and strains caused while working long hours at a laptop or mobile phone. One should stretch out a stiff neck as also give the neck a little rest and relaxation. Alternate Ice and Heat can be applied for neck pain relief. A relaxing massage may help. One can also take Over-the-Counter Pain Relievers. A stiff neck is generally not a cause for alarm. However, **see a doctor if the stiffness is accompanied by other symptoms, such as a fever, a headache, or irritability**. Also see a doctor if the stiffness does not go away within a few days after trying home treatments and gentle stretching.

Some symptoms and Homeopathic medicines to be taken three times a day are given below:

- **Cracking of bone in the neck when moving head.** Cocculus 30.
- **Pain due to injury or strain with stiffness.** Arnica 200 and Bryonia 200.
- **Pain in nape of neck with pain below right shoulder.** Chelidonium 200

**Backache**

Backache is an almost universal problem. But there are different nuances to the pains. Some symptoms and medicines to be taken three times a day are given below:

- **Backache due to injury, old or new.** Arnica 1000 and Hypericum 200.
- **Backache in the region of the kidney or lower back.** Berberis Vulgaris 200 and Calcarea Carb 200.
- **Patient leaning forward due to backache.** Aesculus 200.
- **Backache with stiffness which is better from pressure and worse from movement.** Bryonia 200.
- **Backache with stiffness where patient feels better with motion and lying on a hard bed.** Rhus Tox 200.
- **Backache when bending forward to sweep floor or lift things.** Calcarea Flour 200.
- **Backache which spreads down one or both legs.** Colocynthis 200.

**Pain in Tail Bone**

Pain in tail bone can be due to various reasons. One should buy a scooter tube, inflate it and sit on it to reduce pain. Some symptoms and medicines to be taken two times a day are given below:

- **Due to injury old or recent.** Arnica 1000 and Hypericum 200.
- **When pain is not due to injury.** Conium 200 and Lachesis 200.

**Sciatica**

Abnormal pressure on the sciatica nerve located in the lower back due to deformity in the spine due to injury or posture during work (common among those who work long hours on the computer or lap top) can cause pain in the neck or lower back from where it may run into the legs. The pain may come suddenly or gradually. **Physiotherapy to reduce pressure on the nerve is an important part of the cure. An oil named "Trois" by Venus remedies can be applied on the painful part. The oil can also be used for other pains.** Some symptoms and medicines to be taken two times a day are given below:

- **With sensation of ice water being poured in the part.** Aconite 30.
- **Pain in hip joint and knee.** Colocynthis 200.
- **Pain moving down right thigh.** Dioscorea 30.
- **Pain down left thigh into leg.** Kali Bi 200.
- **Pain like electric flashes and cramps.** Veratrum Alb 200

**Spondylosis**

In spondylosis, the patient has pain and stiffness in the region of the neck. Pain is severe on moving the neck. **An oil called "Trois" by Venus remedies can be applied on the painful region.** Some symptoms and medicines to be taken two times a day are given below:

- **Pain with numbness in feet and legs.** Aconite 30 and Bryonia 200.
- **Pain with numbness of fingers of the hands.** Bryonia 200 and Cimicifuga 200.
- **Pain with spasms or cramps in neck muscles.** Bryonia 200 and Cicuta 200.
- **Pain in neck with pain in right shoulder blade.** Bryonia 200 and Chelidonium 30.

**Tennis elbow**

Tennis elbow is the name given to severe pain in elbow of tennis players and others due to excessive strain. The patient is unable to do anything with that hand. Grandma once suffered from a severe attack of tennis elbow. She could not dress by herself. **One month of treatment at Command Hospital, Kolkata which included daily physiotherapy produced no results. Finally, she went to a "bone setter". He fully cured her with three bandages in three weeks.**

Try Arnica 200 and Ruta G 200, two times a day for a few weeks. If diabetic add Lactic Acid 30. If of right hand try Ferrum Muriticum 30 along with Arnica and Ruta.

**Blisters**

**Blisters on the palm or feet is a common problem with sports persons. If they burst, it can become a nasty painful wound.** Blisters can also be due to insect bites, some illnesses and burns. Blisters should never be punctured with needles.

Some symptoms and Homeopathic medicines are given below:

- **Due to insect bite.** Apis 200.
- **In sports persons or others due to rubbing.** Arnica 200 and Cantharis 200. Also apply Cantharis mother tincture on the blister.
- **If blister bursts and becomes infected and painful.** Arnica 200 and Hepar Sulph 200. If the person is diabetic take Arsenic Alb 200 or 1000 to prevent gangrene from developing.

# 19

# Problems of the Aged

The aged, the so-called senior citizen, have many problems. Blessed are those who live in a joint family among loving children and grand-children, with no financial or health problems. The blessed are a few. **A vast majority is consigned to a lonely existence, often in poverty. Staying healthy is vital for the aged. To stay healthy they must eat healthy, remain active both socially and physically, and tackle medical problems as soon as they appear.** The option of staying at an old age home is better than living alone, though many including Grandpa's mother did not opt for it. Grandpa discusses some health issues of the old in this chapter.

**Dementia and Alzheimer's Disease**

**Dementia is a disease where there is a marked deterioration in the in the intellectual and physical condition of aged persons (usually above 65). There is disorientation of memory. Patient forgets names and recent events but older memories are preserved.** The patient loses sense of time and interest in life. Alzheimer's disease is the most common form of dementia and may contribute to 60-70% of cases. Currently more than 55 million people live with dementia worldwide, and there are nearly 10 million new cases every year. **Dementiais often overlooked in the early stages because the onset is gradual. Common symptoms may include forgetfulness, losing track of the time and becoming lost in familiar places.** As dementia progresses to the middle stage, the signs and symptoms become clearer and may include becoming forgetful of recent events and people's names, becoming confused while at home, having increasing difficulty with communication, needing help with personal care, experiencing behaviour changes, including wandering and repeated questioning. The late stage of dementia is one of near total dependence and inactivity. Memory disturbances are serious and may include becoming unaware of the time and place, having difficulty recognizing relatives and friends, having an increasing need for assisted self-care and having difficulty walking. Some patients can become aggressive.

**Allopathy has no medicine for dementia.** One can reduce their risk of cognitive decline and dementia by remaining physically active, not smoking, avoiding excessive use of alcohol, controlling their weight, eating a healthy diet, and maintaining healthy blood pressure, cholesterol and blood sugar levels. Additional risk factors include depression, social isolation, low educational attainment, cognitive inactivity and air pollution. Some symptoms and Homeopathic medicines are given below:

- **Patient loses his memory, is absent minded, melancholy, easily offended and has cramps in calves.** Two doses of Anacardium 200 and Baryta Carb 200 daily till condition improves.
- **Patient loses his memory, is indifferent to conditions around him and is unable to understand instructions or carryon conversation.** Two doses of Phosphoric Acid 30 daily till conditions improve.

- **Loss of memory, mental weakness, irresolute, loss of confidence, confused and shy. Aversion to strangers.** Baryt Carb 200.
- **The patient has great mental and physical depression. Loss of memory. No interest in life. Has nightmares.** Kali Phos 30
- **Complete loss of mental faculties. Unable to understand or appreciate own suffering. Thinks he is not at home.** Opium 200.
- **Mental debility is followed by physical debility. Partial loss of memory. Comprehension is weakened. Cannot find the right word. Has difficulty in conversing.** Phosphoric Acid 30.
- **Loss of memory, low spirit, restless, fidgety, over sensitive to what others say with an exaggerated idea of one's importance. Dread of death when left alone.** Phosphorous 200.

**Irritable**

**Some old persons seem always angry and irritable.** They can be mean and spiteful. They cannot tolerate themselves and also others. Give one dose of Chamomilla 200 three times a day till temper is under control.

**Melancholy**

Some common symptoms and medicines which are to be taken three times a day are given below:

- **Dreads people and desires to be alone. Intensely shy. Loss of love of life. Music irritates. Dwells on unpleasant things.** Ambra Grisea 200.
- **Sits in a stupid manner. Notices nothing. Aimless wandering from home. Cursing or howling at night.** Veratrum Alb 200.

**Memory Loss**

Like all other faculties, old people tend to lose their memory. Some common symptoms and medicines which are to be taken are given below

- **Unable to remember names.** Anacardium 200 and Lycopodium 200, two times a day for a month.
- **Unable to recognize localities or find one's house.** Glonoine 200.

**Cataract**

Cataract is a common problem in the aged. Surgery is usually necessary to replace the lens. **One needs to go to a doctor who does such operations every day.** Only one eye should be operated at a time. These operations are not always successful. Grandpa's father lost eyesight in both eyes after cataract operations. The medical science has improved a lot since then. One must get the operation done at a well-known clinic. **Never get both eyes operated together. After-operation care is very important and precautions recommended by the doctor must be taken faithfully.**

If detected in early stages, treatment under Homeopathy is possible. But the patient must go to an established doctor or Homeopathic Hospital.

**Glaucoma**

**This is another eye problem which effects the aged. There is a progressive loss of vision with increased pressure inside the eye ball.** The pressure causes pain and blurring of vision. One must consult an eye specialist as early as possible. Some symptoms and medicines to be taken three times a day are given below:

- **Pain in the eye. A green halo is seen around light at night.** Osmium 30.
- **Dim vision. Momentary loss of vision as from fainting. Objects look red.** Phosphorous 200.

**Problems of the Retina**

**There are two kinds of problems, detachment and haemorrhage. Both are very serious problems and can lead to blindness. One must see a specialist as early as possible.** Retinal detachment is usually a result of aging. It can also be due to injury. Risk of retinal detachment increases with age, family history, cataract operation and severe myopia or near sightedness. **The main symptoms are seeing flashes of light in the corners of the eye, increase in the number and size of floaters, darkening of peripheral vision (side vision) and darkening or loss of vision in one portion of the eye.** Retinal detachment is usually painless. If the above symptoms appear, one must immediately see a specialist. Also avoid lifting heavy things, avoid jerks which are unavoidable when riding a motorcycle or scooter and even a car on unpaved roads or roads with pothole and speed breakers.

Some symptoms and Homeopathic medicines to be taken two times a day are:

- **Seeing flashes of light. Sudden loss of part vision.** Argentum Nitricum 200 and Aurum Met 200.
- **Detachment due to injury.** Arnica 200 or 1000 and Gelsemium 200.
- **Sudden dimming of vision. Black floaters. Patient has Myiopia or double vision.** Argentum Nitricum 200 and Gelsemium 200.
- **Retinal haemorrhage.** Borothrops 30. Twice a day for 7 days.

**Loss of Hearing**

Age results in loss of hearing in many. Some common symptoms and medicines which are to be taken are given below. If improvement is not there one should go for a hearing aid.

- **Loss of hearing in one ear.** Ambra Grisea 30.
- **Finds difficulty in hearing human voice but not other sounds. Hears echoes.** Phosphorous 200 till improvement is seen or a week.
- **Hardness of hearing with crackling sound.** Baryta Carb 200.

**Weak Heart**

**Heart problem is characterized by breathlessness, slow pulse and palpitations. There is weakness. Even a short walk can be tiring.** There may be pain in left shoulder or elbow. The problems are of two types. Weak pulse may indicate the need to have a pacemaker. High pulse rate may indicate the need to have stents inserted into blocked arteries or even a bypass operation. One should have an instrument which can measure blood pressure and pulse at home and monitor blood pressure and pulse particularly if not feeling well. **One must consult a heart specialist and get prescribed tests done.** Some Homeopathic medicines which can be used in not so serious cases are given below:

- **Blood pressure is high. There could be pain in the chest.** Veratrum Viride 30.
- **Blood pressure low, pulse is feeble, volent palpitation with loss of balance and gas. There may be chest pain.** Cactus 30.
- **Violent palpitation. Palpitation from least activity.** Belladona 200.
- **Palpitation with irregular and rapid pulse.** Veratrum Alb 200.
- **Crataegus 200 can be taken once a week as a tonic by those who get tired easily.**
- **Digitalis 30 can be taken once a week as a tonic by persons with slow irregular pulse, numb fingers and cold feet.**

**Asthma Bronchial**

First Aid as explained in Chapter on First Aid. Aged patients with no strength or vitality should be administered Carbo Veg 200 four times a day.

**Asthma Cardiac**

**Cardiac Asthma is a disease of the aged. Attacks usually come at night.** First aid is the same as for bronchial asthma. **The Patient must be taken to a hospital at the earliest possible.** Some common symptoms and medicines which are to be taken three times a day by not so serious patients are given below:

- **With high blood pressure.** Baryta Mur 200.
- **With weak pulse and weak heart.** Digitalis 30.

**Coughs and Colds**

**Chronic cold in aged persons is a common complaint. Such persons must be given Carbo Veg 200 two times a day for months and, if necessary, years.** Some additional symptom-based medicines to be taken two times a day are:

- **With rattling sound during breathing.** Antim Tart 200.
- **With weak lung power.** Bacillium 200.
- **With thick yellow sputum which is difficult to take out.** Hydrastatis 200.

**Problems with Digestion and Stool**

- **Indigestion.** Abies Nigera 200.
- **Diarrhoea or constipation due to over eating or indiscriminate eating.** Antim Crud 200.
- **Weak digestion.** Baryta Carb 200.
- **Lack of appetite, acidity, gas problem.** Carbo Veg 200.
- **Constipation. Stool is hard and dry.** Sulphur 200 and Bryonia 200
- **Frequent desire. Only a little stool passes at a time.** Nux Vom 200.
- **First hard and then gushing. Flatulence.** Lycopodium 200.
- **Involuntary passing of stool. Diarrhoea.** Apis 200.
- **Involuntary, unnoticed but solid.** Aloe 200.
- **Copious, watery, gushing out with gas. Early morning.** Croton Tig 200.
- **Unsure whether wind or stool will come out.** Aloe 200

**Prostrate Problems**

Prostrate problems are quite common among the aged male. The prostate gland gets enlarged. The symptoms relate mainly to passage of urine. (Also see under "Male Sexual Problems"). Some symptoms and medicines to be taken three times a day are given below:

- **Enlargement and indurations of prostrate. Urine comes in dribble. It starts and stops and restarts. There could be pain. Better witting. Worse walking.** Conium 200
- **Hypertrophy of prostrate. Renewed straining and dribbling after passing urine. Numbness in penis after urination.** Baryta Carb 200.
- **Prostatitis itching and painful irritation of urethra from end of penis to neck of bladder.** Chimaphila 30.
- **Patient with weak heart, low pulse rate, low blood pressure having prostrate problems. Urination difficult. Dribbling discharge. Pain in region of bladder while urinating.** Digitalis 30 and Morphinum 30.
- **Urine falls vertically without any force.** Hepar Sulph 200.

- **Frequent passing of copious urine, particularly at night.** Staphysagria 200.

**Other Urinary Problems**

Some common urinary problems faced by the aged and their medicines to be taken three times a day are given below:

- **Involuntary Discharge. Particularly at night.** Secale 30 and Apis 200.
- **Dribbling. Urine starts and stops again and drips.** Conium 200.
- **Bladder difficulties. Difficulty in passing urine.** No force. Hepar Sulph 200.
- **Inability to pass urine.** Aconite 30 and Camphor 30. One must take patient to the doctor as early as possible.

**Parkinson's Disease**

**Parkinson's diseaseis a long-term degenerative disorder of the central nervous system that mainly affects our limbs. The symptoms usually emerge slowly. The most obvious early symptoms are involuntary shaking of head or limbs, rigidity, slowness of movement and difficulty with walking.** There could be weakening of facial muscles resulting in a vacant look. The head may nod rhythmically.The shaking or rigidity symptoms of the disease result from the death of cells in mid brain. Those with an affected family member are at an increased risk of getting the disease, with certain genes known to be inheritable risk factors. Other risk factors are those who have been exposed to certain pesticides and head injuries. Coffee and tea drinkers are at a reduced risk. Parkinson's disease typically occurs in people over the age of 60. Males are more often affected than females. The average life expectation after diagnosis is between 7 and 15 years. There is no cure for Parkinsons Disease in Allopathy. Treatment aims to reduce the effects of the symptoms.

**There are four symptoms of Parkinsons disease; shaking of head or limbs, slowness of movement, rigidity, and postural instability. The most common early symptom is slow shaking of the hand at rest.** It typically appears in only one hand, eventually affecting both hands as the disease progresses. There may also be involuntary shaking of the head. Rigidity is stiffness in muscles and difficulty in limb movement caused by excessive and continuous contraction of muscles. Rigidity may be associated with joint pain; such pain being a frequent initial manifestation of the disease.

In early stages of Parkinsons Disease, stiffness often tends to affect the neck and shoulder muscles prior to the muscles of the face and extremities. With advancement of the disease, stiffness typically affects the whole body and reduces the ability to move. Postural instability is common in the later stages of the disease. Instability is often absent in the initial stages. A slurred, monotonous, quiet voice, lack of facial expression and difficulty in handwriting are other indications.

**Adequate physical exercise in middle age may reduce the risk of Parkinsons Disease later in life. Coffee and tea drinking also appears to reduce risk.Aging Adults with Parkinson's should avoid high-protein foods**. Dairy products, processed foods, **h**ard-to-chew foods, salty foods like salted cashew or peanuts and bacon, acidic foods like pickles should be avoided. Eating plenty of whole foods, such as **fruits and vegetables, lean protein, beans and legumes, and whole grains**, and staying hydrated are key ways to stay energized and healthy overall. **Fish, monosaturated fatty acids, low levels of dairy, meat and poultry should be part of the diet. Low to moderate alcohol consumption is all right.** Deficiency in B1 (thiamine), B6 (pyridoxine), B9 (folate), or B12 (cobalamin) in particular have been linked to Parkinson's Disease. Patients should take these medicines as supplements.

Some common symptoms and Homeopathic medicines to be taken three times a day till cured are given below. One can also take Hypericum 200 and Opium 200 with the medicines given below.

- **Constant nodding of the head.** Aurum Sulph 30.
- **Involuntary jerking of limbs.** Mag Phos 200.
- **Inability to hold anything in the hands.** Phosphorous 200.

**Arthritis Gout**

Arthritis Gout is a painful inflammation of joints on account of deposit of uric acid in joints. Knees, elbows, wrists or ankles can be affected. See Chapter 21.

**Staggering**

A person is said to be staggering when he lacks coordination during walking. Some common symptoms and medicines which are to be taken are given below

- **There is loss of balance.** Administer Conium 200, twice a day.

- **Vertigo on rising from seat or bed.** Phosphorous 200.

**Sleep**

Some common symptoms and medicines which are to be taken are given below

- **Great drowsiness in old people. Specially after meals. Lascivious dreams.** Phosphorus 200.
- **Cannot sleep from worry. Must get up. Anxious dreams.** Ambra Grisea 30.

**Conclusion**

Problems of old age are numerous and gets worse as we age. However, old people need to learn to die with dignity and not allow too much money to be spent on their treatment. Homeopathy provides cheap and effective treatment for most problems of the aged.

**Grandpa is 82 years old and believes that most of his vital organs have suffered some wear and tear.** To avoid further detritions of the organs and faculties, I have decided to take six pills of one medicine as a preventive on empty stomach every morning. The sequence is as under:

- Day 1. Baryta Carb 200. Improves memory and reduces chance of dementia.
- Day 2. Calcarea Carb 200. Delays cataract, back ache and rheumatic pains.
- Day 3. Berberis Vulgaris 200. Backache, helps functioning of kidney, liver and gall bladder.
- Day 4. Chelidonium 30. Improves functioning of liver and gallbladder.
- Day 5. Phosphorus 200. Delays cataract, improves functioning of liver, strengthens bones, improves liver functions and improves hearing.
- Day 6. Anacardium 200. Removes depression and improves memory.
- Day 7. Conium 200. Improves functioning ofheart and postrate. In case of women, Conium should be replaced by Baryta Carb 200 which reduces degenerative changes in the functioning of brain, lungs and heart

**One may devise a different set of medicines based on their medical problems.** For example, for Grandma who has diabetes, joint pains and breathlessness, Grandpa has given her a different set of medicines as under.

- Day 1. Arsenic Alb 200. Medicine for diabetes and respiratory problems like breathlessness. Also improves functioning of heart.
- Day 2. Calcarea Carb 200. Delays cataract, back ache and rheumatic pains.
- Day 3. Berberis Vulgaris 200. Backache, helps functioning of kidney, liver and gall bladder.
- Day 4. Chelidonium 30. Improves functioning of liver and gallbladder.
- Day 5. Baryta Carb 200. Helps improve memory.
- Day 6. Calcarea Carb 200. Improves functioning of liver, digestive system and strengthens constitution.
- Day 7. Calcarea Flour 200. Helps in varicose veins and back pain.

**No book suggests this line of treatment. Grandpa has tried this for over ten years without any problems and intends to continue**. After angioplasty in 2005, Grandpa takes six Allopathic pills every day. Grandma has been taking four allopathic pills and insulin before going to sleep every day for diabetes, blood pressure and other problems. **Grandpa does not think there is any problem if one takes one Homeopathic medicine a day to keep the doctor away.**

# 20
# Problem Of Children

Children sometimes suffer from diseases which are not common among adults. The dosage of medicines of **children below 12 should be half the standard adult does of four pills and three instead of six pills where six have been recommended.**

**Adenoids**

Adenoid is a pad of tissue that lies at the back of the nose close to the mouth cavity. When inflamed or enlarged, it makes it difficult for the child to breathe. The child gets tired easily and shuns physical activity. He may suffer from blocked nose and middle ear pain. The treatment should start with one dose of Bacillinum 200 which should be repeated if required after two weeks. Next, the patient should be given two doses of Silicea 200 for 2 days to cure pus if any. This should be followed with one of the following medicines two times a day till the nose block is removed:

- **When there is pain in the ear:** Agraphis Nutans 30
- **When the child is fat and tonsils are swollen**: Calcarea Carb 30
- **When the child is thin and tonsils are swollen**: Calcarea Phos 30

**Bed Wetting**

A child sometimes wets the bed and feels ashamed. He should not be rebuked. Some common symptoms and medicines to be taken two times a day are:

- **Urine is foul smelling and stains the bed sheet.** Benzoic Acid 30.
- **Bedwetting without waking up**. Belladona 30.
- **Bed wetting before midnight.** Causticum 30.

### Common Cold

This is a very common disease. Some common symptoms and medicines to be taken two times a day are:

- **With light fever and headache.** Aconite 30. Can repeat dose once every hour till fever goes.
- **With violent cough. Face turns red.** Belladonna 30.
- **With dry cough. There may be pain in chest.** Aconite 30 and Bryonia 200.
- **Due to getting wet in rains.** Dulcamara 30.
- **With wheezing and difficult breathing. The chest is full of mucus.** Aconite 30 and Ipecac 30.
- **When there is a lot of mucus but it does not come out.** Antim Tart 200.
- **With green stringy mucus which is difficult to take out.** Kali BI 30.
- **Non-stop flow of thin mucus.** Merc Sol 30.
- **Nose blocked. Dry cough.** Nux Vom 30.
- **With bland yellow or green mucus.** Loose cough. Pulsatilla 30.
- **Breathlessness. Exhausting cough. Pain right side of chest.** Cheledonium 30.

### Chicken Pox

The disease starts with a slight fever. Eruptions appear on the second day, Pus forms in the eruptions. Eruptions dry up after six to seven days and the scales fall off. There is itching. Child is irritable and has poor appetite. The treatment should start with one dose of Variolinum 200. No other medicine for 24 hours. Antim Tart 30 four times a day till fever subsides. Rhus Tox 30, three times a day to reduce itching. Merc Sol 30 once a day for three days after fever subsides.

### Dentition Problems

Some common symptoms and medicines to be taken three times a day are:

- **Teeth decay as soon as they appear.** Kreosote 30.
- **Diarrhoea during dentition.** Podophyllum 30.

### German Measles

It is a minor disease. Rashes appear on the face in the form of red spots on the first day. Rashes spread all over the body on the second day and start disappearing on the third. Some common symptoms and medicines to be taken two times a day are:

- **Fever with restlessness.** Aconite 30.
- **Sore throat and enlarged glands.** Belladonna 30 to be taken alternately with Aconite 30.
- **Fever with Chill and sweats.** Ferrum Phos 30.
- **Child weepy. Wants company and sympathy. Cold is a predominant symptom.** Pulsatilla 30.

**Nappy Rash**

Apply Calendula ointment or mother tincture.

**Night Terrors**

Child wakes up suddenly in great fear. He screams or mumbles in sleep. Give one dose of Aconite 30 followed by Belladona 30.

**Nose Bleed**

Some common symptoms and medicines to be taken two times a day are:

- **Due to injury.** Arnica 200.
- **Bleeding drop by drop.** Hamamelis 30.
- **For no apparent reason.** Millefolium 30.

**Phimosis**

Phimosis is a disease where tight foreskin causes problems during urination. Some common symptoms and medicines which are to be taken two times a day are given below:

- **Sudden occurrence.** Aconite 30.
- **With swelling, soreness and burning below the foreskin.** One dose of Apis 200 followed by Nitric Acid 30.

**Constipation**

Treatment should start with one dose of Sulphur 200. Some common symptoms and medicines to be taken two times a day are given below:

- Infants during dentition. Magnesia Mur 200 and Silicia 200.
- Obstinate constipation in children. Paraffine 30 and Sepia 200.

### Pneumonia

**Pneumonia is a dangerous disease of the lungs and the child needs to be taken to a doctor as early as possible.** The main symptoms are high temperature, cold with or without cough, shivering, rapid and heavy breathing and at times vomiting and convulsions. **Whether confirmed or not, as soon as the above symptoms are seen, give one dose of Aconite 30 every hour for 24 hours and one dose of Sulphur 30 every alternate day along with selected medicine.** Some common symptoms and additional medicines to be taken two times a day are:

- **Sharp pain in centre of chest.** Bryonia 200.
- **Breathlessness. Exhausting cough. Pain right side of chest.** Cheledonium 30.
- **Exhausting suffocating cough.** Nausea. Ipecac 30
- **Breathing difficult. Pain under breast bone. Rust coloured sputa.** Phosphorous 200.

### Rickets

Rickets is a common problem in children from very poor families due to malnourishment. Bones are soft, bent and malformed. Forehead is very prominent. The child reaches tenth month without cutting teeth. Improved diet and a calcium tonic will help the child. Some common symptoms and medicines to be taken two times a day are:

- **Head and joints enlarged. Teeth decaying. Belly swollen.** Calcarea Carb 30.
- **Similar symptoms but diarrhoea is dominating.** Calcarea Phos 30.

### Sore Throat

Some common symptoms and medicines to be taken two times a day are:

- **Throat red and inflamed. Tonsils swollen. Pain while swallowing.** Belladonna 30.
- **Throat sore on taking very cold drinks.** Bryonia 30.
- **Pain is severe. Pus in tonsil.** Hepar Sulph 200
- **Pus in tonsil but pain is mild.** Merc Sol. 30
- **Throat purple. Swallowing very painful. Worse left side.** Lachesis 30.

- **Takes cold easily. Tonsils swollen and painful. Swallowing painful. Voice hoarse.** Baryta Carb 200.

**Stomach Upsets**

Some common symptoms and medicines to be taken two times a day are:

- **Troubles due to over eating. Tongue white coated. Foul eructation. Stomach pains when pressed.** Antim Crud 200.
- **Children's diarrhoea. Abdomen gurgles and rumbles.** Veratrun Alb 200 and China 200.
- **Food poisoning.** Arsenic Alb 200.
- **No appetite. Pain in the centre of stomach just below rib cage radiating in all directions.** Argentum Nitricum 200.
- **With nausea and vomiting.** Ipecac 30.
- **Stomach upset due to excessive heavy fatty food.** Pulsatilla 30.
- **Rice water like loose motions.** Veratrum Alb 200

**Tonsillitis**

Swollen tonsils are accompanied by high temperature, white coated tongue, dry cough and bad breath. The problem is common in children. Some common symptoms and medicines which are to be taken two times a day are given below:

- **Sudden attack due to exposure to cold air.** Aconite 30
- **Swelling is the main symptom.** Apis 200.
- **Tonsils enlarged and fiery red. Difficulty is swallowing. Worse right side.** Belladonna 200.
- **Pain worse on left side.** Lachesis 200.
- **Pus but without shooting pain. Voice affected. Fever with chill and sweat. Worse at night and in bed.** Merc Sol 200.
- **Tonsils swollen and painful. Swallowing painful. Voice hoarse.** Baryta Carb 200.
- **Chronic cases where patient has frequent attacks or suffers for a long time.** Silicea 200.

**Worms**

This is a common problem with kids. Some symptoms which indicate presence of worms in the child are picking at the nose, grinding of teeth when sleeping, impaired appetite, straining at stool and itching and irritation around the anus. Give Cina 30 two times a day for two weeks. Cina 200 should be given to children over 10 years.

**Under Developed Infants**

If an infant does not develop properly, if his bones do not grow administer two pills of Calcarea Carb 30 and Sulphur 30 three times a day for a month.

**Stoppage of urine in babies**

A new-born may not pass urine due to shock during birth. Give two pills of Aconite 30 and the problem may be solved.

**Child Sensitive to Pain**

If a child is peevish and extremely sensitive to pain and keeps crying, give Chamomilla 30, three times a day for a week.

**Conclusion**

When Grandpa's children were small, he often took them to Homeopathic doctors for treatment. However, one should not be very rigid about it. **Do take them to a practicing doctor for serious problems like high fevers or pneumonia.**

# 21

# Arthritis, Gout and Rehumatism

**Arthritis**

**Arthritis is a joint disorder featuring inflammation of one or more joints.** It can be caused by injury (leading to osteoarthritis), metabolic abnormalities (such as gout), hereditary factors, the direct and indirect effect of infections (bacterial and viral), and a misdirected system with autoimmunity (such as in rheumatoid arthritis). Arthritis can affect men and women, children and adults. Approximately 350 million people worldwide have arthritis. More than 27 million Americans have osteoarthritis. Approximately 1.3 million Americans suffer from rheumatoid arthritis. More than half of those with arthritis are under 65 years of age.

**Diets does not play a major in precipitating or exacerbating arthritis. However, oils of fish have been shown to have anti-inflammatory properties. Some patients benefit from omega-3 fatty acid supplements.**

**Treatments available include physio-therapy, splinting, cold-pack application, paraffin wax dips, anti-inflammatory medications, pain medications, immune-altering medications, and surgical operations or joint replacement surgery. Ayurveda have some oils which can help reduce pain and restore ligaments in joints. Grandma applies "Doctor Ortho" oil on her knee every day after bath.**

Some symptoms and medicines to be taken two times a day are given below:

- **Pain in joints and bones:** Causticum 200 and Eupatorium Perf 200.
- **Pain increases with movement:** Bryonia 200

- **Pain decreases with movement:** Rhus Tox 200

- **In diabetic patients.** Arsenic Alb 200 and Lactic Acid 200.
- **Arthritis of small joints in hands, fingers and toes.** Actea Spicata 30 and Pulsatilla 30.
- **When knee joints are the main problem.** Calcarea Flour 200 and Sticta 200.
- **When the main problem is pain in bones.** Eupator Perf 200 and Causticum 200.

**Gout**

**Gout is a disease that results from an overload of uric acid in the body. This overload of uric acid leads to the formation of tiny crystals of urate that deposit in tissues of the body, especially the joints.** When crystals form in the joints, it causes recurring attacks of joint inflammation (arthritis). Gout is considered a chronic and progressive disease. **Chronic gout can also lead to deposits of hard lumps of uric acid in the tissues, particularly in and around the joints and may cause joint destruction, decreased kidney function, and lead to kidney stone.**

Gouty arthritis is typically an extremely painful attack with a rapid onset of joint inflammation. The joint inflammation is precipitated by deposits of uric acid crystals in the joint fluid (synovial fluid) and joint lining (synovial lining). Intense joint inflammation occurs as the immune system reacts, causing white blood cells to engulf the uric acid crystals and chemical messengers of inflammation to be released, leading to pain, heat, and redness of the joint tissues. As gout progresses, the attacks of gouty arthritis typically occur more frequently and often in additional joints.

**The small joint at the base of the big toe is the most common site of an acute gout attack of arthritis.** Other joints that are commonly affected include the ankles, knees, wrists, fingers, and elbows. Acute gout attacks are characterized by a rapid onset of pain in the affected joint followed by warmth, swelling, reddish discoloration, and marked tenderness. **Tenderness can be intense so that even a blanket touching the skin over the affected joint can be unbearable.** Patients can develop fever with the acute gout attacks. These painful attacks usually subside in hours to days, with or without medication. In rare instances, an attack can last for weeks. Most patients with gout will experience repeated attacks of arthritis over the years. Gout usually attacks one joint at a time, while other arthritis conditions and rheumatoid arthritis, usually attack multiple joints simultaneously.

**Gout is clearly diet-related. Foods that are high in proteins, especially red meats and shellfish, can worsen the condition.** In addition, certain foods increase the levels of uric acid, including alcohol (especially beer) and those foods containing high amounts of fructose (such as the corn syrup found in soft drinks). Gluten-containing foods (wheat, barley, rye) can worsen joint pains in some patients

**Gout can be controlled by maintaining adequate fluid intake, reducing weight, dietary changes to reduce protein intake, reducing alcohol consumption and taking medications to lower the uric acid level in the blood.**

Maintaining adequate fluid intake helps prevent acute gout attacks. Adequate fluid intake also decreases the risk of kidney stone formation in patients with gout. Alcohol is known to have diuretic effects that can contribute to dehydration and precipitate acute gout attacks. **Alcohol has two major effects that worsen gout.** It slows down the excretion of uric acid from the kidneys and causes dehydration. Both contribute to the precipitation of uric acid crystals in the joints.

**Dietary changes can help reduce uric acid levels in the blood.** Persons having signs of gout must avoid shellfish and organ meats such as liver, brains, kidneys, and sweetbreads. Red meat or seafood consumption increases the risk of gout attacks, while dairy food consumption seemed to reduce the risk. Vegetable consumption does not aggravate gout. Weight reduction can be helpful in lowering the risk of recurrent attacks of gout. This is best accomplished by reducing dietary fat and calorie intake, combined with a regular exercise program.

Some Homeopathic medicines for Gout are:

- **To reduce uric acid in blood:** Benzoic Acid 200
- **Shooting pain and redness of joints:** Aconite Ferox 30
- **Chronic gout, toe and fingers contracted:** Lycopodium 200
- **Big toe swollen. Pain rises from lower to upper parts of body:** Ledum 200

**Rheumatism or Rheumatoid Arthritis**

**Rheumatoid arthritis isan autoimmune and inflammatory disease.** Here, the body's immune system attacks healthy cells in the body by mistake, and causes inflammation (painful swelling) in the affected parts of the body. Rheumatism mainly attacks the joints. It usually attacks many joints at once. No one knows why it happens. The first sign of rheumatoid arthritis is extreme tiredness and lack of energy. There may be slight fever. There may be unexplained weight loss. Joints could be stiff, tender and painful. There may be swelling and redness of the joint. Over long periods of time, the inflammation associated with rheumatoid arthritis can cause bone erosion and joint deformity. **While there's no cure for rheumatoid arthritis in allopathy, physiotherapy and medication can help slow the disease's progression. It is a serious medical problem and every effort needs to be made to contain the ill effects.** Rheumatism is similar to Arthritis except that the patient may have fever and pain is not only in joints but also in muscles and tendons. Some symptoms and medicines to be taken two times a day are given below:

- **When the pains start from the feet and rise upwards.** Ledum Pal 200.
- **When large muscles like thighs are affected.** Cimicifuga 200.
- **When fever is persistent.** Formic Acid 30.
- **Pain comes suddenly. Joints red, hot and sensitive.** Belladonna 200.
- **Pain comes slowly and gradually increases in severity. Better from pressure, lying on painful side and rest.** Bryonia 200.
- **Pain in neck, back and thighs. Relief from motion.** Rhus Tox 200.
- **Pain in thigh and right hip joint.** Chelidonium 30.
- **Pain in left hip joint.** Stramonium 30.
- **Rheumatic pain in joints, particularly ankle:** Argentum Metalicum 200
- **Rheumatic pain in small joints and wrist, fingers, and toes:** Actaea Spicata 30
- **Violent pain in muscles, better by warm application:** Mag Phos 200 and Calcarea Carb 30.
- **Pain in knees, ankles, small joints and feet. Pain shifts from limb to limb**. Pulsatilla 30.
- **There is fever and severe pain in cervical bones, shoulders and joints.** Veratrum Viride 30

**Vitamin D is beneficial for those suffering from rheumatic arthritis.** Doctor may be approached to prescribe medication. **One should also spend at least 30 minutes in the sun, before 10 AM or after 4 PM.** One can also get more vitamin D by taking certain types of fish, such as salmon and mackerel, egg yolks, cheese, and liver.

**Lifestyle changes and home remedies including homeopathy are the only ways to cope with rheumatic arthritis.** One must exercise regularly. Gentle exercise can help strengthen the muscles around your joints, and it can help reduce fatigue one might feel. One should consult a physiotherapist. One can apply heat or cold or both alternately. Heat and cold can help ease one's pain and relax painful muscles and joints. One must also try to change one's lifestyle and find ways to cope with pain by reducing stress.

# 22

# Treatment of Cancers

**Cancer is a dreaded disease and requires specialist treatment at a cancer hospital. It can be quick acting and kill in a few months or slow acting and kill in a few years.** It is a curse of God or Man when we consider that products of human greed like carcinogen pesticides enter the food chain and human habits like smoking and tobacco chewing cause cancer. Its treatment is not available in many towns of India. **Early detection gives some chance of success. Late detection is a death sentence.** Sudden unexplained loss of weight is usually the first warning signal and must be thoroughly investigated. **Prevention of cancer has been discussed in Chapter 6: Prevention of diseases.**

Naturopathy and Homeopathy claim to be able to cure some types of cancers. **Grandpa has no first-hand knowledge if they work. However, a drowning man will clutch at any straw. Grandpa would like to inform his readers of what Homeopathy has to offer towards treating cancer.** Homeopathic medicines can be taken along with any allopathic formulations prescribed by giving a gap of one hour between Homeopathic and Allopathic medicines.

**Cancer of the Mouth**

Cancer of the mouth can be on the lips, tongue, gum, palate or on the lining of the cheek. They are in the form of small, red, hard tumours or lesions which do not heal. Surgery and radiation therapy is effective for lip cancer but difficult for other forms of cancer of the mouth.

**Cancer of the lips**

Hydrastatis mother tincture should be applied. Some common symptoms and medicines to be taken two times a day are:

- **Lips bluish with coppery eruptions.** Aurum Ars 200.
- **Hard tumour of the lip.** Conium 1000.
- **Ulcers and lesions on the lip.** Condurango 30.

**Cancer of the tongue**

Some common symptoms and medicines to be taken two times a day are:

- **Tongue dry, swollen, inflamed, ulcerated. Unable to swallow.** Apis 1000.
- **Tongue red, sore, bleeds. So swollen that it fills the mouth.** Crotalus H 200.

**Cancer of the Throat**

**Cancer of the throat attacks the sound box and vocal cords. There is persistent soreness of the throat and difficulty in swallowing solid food.** There may be pain in ears and throat. There is loss of weight. Some common symptoms and medicines to be taken two times a day are:

- **Dirty looking growth in the throat.** Arsenic Alb 200.
- **Continuous dry hacking cough.** Conium 1000
- **Fibrous growth in the throat. Glands swollen. Pain at the root of the tongue extending to the ears.** Phytolacca 200.

**Cancer of the Lungs**

**In the early stages there is persistent dry cough. There is difficult breathing and gradual loss of weight. Later there is pain in the chest and difficulty in swallowing.** Carbo Veg 200 should be given three times a day. Some common symptoms and additional medicines to be taken two times a day are:

- **Coughing pure blood.** Millefolium 200.
- **Sputum a mixture of blood and mucus.** Phosphorus 200.
- **Violent cough with thick, yellow mucus but no blood.** Silicea 200.

**Cancer of the Food Pipe**

This is very difficult to detect in the early stages. **The main symptoms are pain in the food pipe, loss of weight and choking while drinking liquids.** The medicine is Arsenic Alb 200, to be taken two times a day.

**Cancer of the Stomach**

This is also very difficult to detect in the early stages. **The main symptoms are slow and steady loss of weight, loss of appetite, anaemia, pain in upper abdomen, vomiting blood or blood in stool.** The main medicines are Phosphorus 10000 once a week and Cabo Veg 200 to be taken 3 times a day. Some common symptoms and additional medicines to be taken two times a day are:

- **Blood in stool or vomit.** Millefollium 200.
- **Pain and vomit of food.** Condurango 30.
- **Vomiting of bloody, slimy coffee coloured slime. Sinking feeling in the stomach,** Crotalus H 200.
- **Burning pain, great thirst and inability to retain food,** Nitric Acid 200

**Cancer of the Breast**

**Women run a risk of developing breast cancer between the ages of 45 to 65.** It usually appears as a hard lump in the breast and spreads to the lymph glands in the arm pit and then through the body. The nipple retracts. The skin may ulcerate and become painful. There may be discharge from the nipples. Most can be cured if detected early by operating and removing the affected breast. My mother had the operation and lives problem free even 20 years after the operation. **In Homeopathic treatment Conium 1000 should be given once a day. Phytolacca mother tincture should be applied externally on the breast and armpit for relief from pain.** Some common symptoms and additional medicines to be taken two times a day are:

- **Severe burning in the breast. Great restlessness.** Arsenic Alb 200.
- **Ulceration of the skin of the breast. Acute pain. Armpit glands swollen and hard. Worse left side.** Asterius Rubens 30.
- **Painful tumour in women with very large breasts.** Chimaphilla 30.
- **Breasts hard, painful and purple. Glands in arm pits enlarged. Hard, irregular tumour with retracted nipples.** Phytolacca 200.

**Cancer of the Bowels**

Cancer of the bowels is difficult to detect. **Some symptoms are constipation alternating with mucus, difficulty in passing stool and blood in stool. There is severe pain in the rectum when sitting.** Ruta 1000 is a useful medicine in cancer of lower bowel.

**Cancer of Uterus, Cervix**

**Women between the ages of 40 to 70 are more prone to develop these problems. The warning signals are bleeding from vagina after inter course, unusually heavy periods, flow of blood between periods and post menopause bleeding.** Any unusual bleeding from the vagina requires immediate and proper investigation. **If there is any problem in the uterus after the reproductive phase of life of a woman is over, the uterus should be removed through operation. It ensures a healthy a problem free life.** If for any reason operation is not possible, **Homeopathic medicines can be tried. 10 drops of Caltha Palustris 30 should be given to the patient four times a day.** Some common symptoms and additional medicines to be taken three times a day are:

- **Irregular menstruation. Eruptions on the vulva with itching. Increased sexual desire.** Aurum Arsenic 200.
- **Severe pain which moves down into the thighs.** Carbo Animalis 200.
- **With offensive discharge, bleeding and pain.** Carsiniosin 200.
- **Oozing blood with terrible colour.** Kreosote 30
- **Tumour in uterus.** Kali Iod 30.

**Cancer of Ovary**

**There are no symptoms till the cancer is in an advanced stage. The main symptoms are low back pain, unusual vaginal bleeding and swelling of abdomen with pain and growth which can be felt in the pelvis. Removal through surgery is the best option.** Removal of one ovary does not affect child bearing capability. My wife had one ovary removed as a teenager before marriage. She bore me two children. Some common symptoms and medicines to be taken two times a day are:

- **Severe pain from hip to knee. Worse on the right side.** Kali Carb 30.
- **Pain and swelling on the left side**. Lacesis 200.

**Cancer of the Prostrate**

Prostrate operation is dangerous and success rate is not very high. **The medicine for prostate cancer is Conium 1000 once a day, Baryta Carb 200 and Crotalus H 200 two times a day.** The medicine for cancer of male genitals is Conium 1000 once a day and Arsenic Alb 1000 three times a day.

**Cancer of the Blood or Leukaemia**

**Leukaemia is production of abnormal white cells which over power the other element of the blood. The symptoms are anaemia, loss of weight, weakness, swelling of spleen, liver and lymph nodes and persistent low fever.** Chances of survival are not very bright. The recommended medicines are Ferrum Aceticum 1000 or 10000 once a day and Picric Acid 30 and Iridium 30 two times a day.

**Cancer of the Bone**

**This is also very difficult to detect. The main symptoms are severe and continuous pain in a bone which does not respond to Eupator Perf 200 or allopathic pain killers.** Some common symptoms and medicines to be given are given below.

- **If the bone affected is of the lower jaw or tibia,** give Phosphorus 1000 two times a day.
- **If there is burning pain in the bone** give Euphorbium 200, two times a day or as required to relieve the suffering of the patient.
- **Pains at night with a sensation of bones being scraped.** Phosphoric Acid 200, two times a day or as required to relieve the suffering of the patient.

**Pain Killers for Cancer Patients**

Some common symptoms and medicines to be taken two times a day or as otherwise indicated or as necessary are:

- **Stinging pain, intolerance of heat and the slightest touch.** Apis 1000.
- **Cutting pain in breast cancer.** Asterious Rubens 200.
- **Burning pains. Nightly aggravation. Restlessness and exhaustion.** Arsenic Alb 200 and Euphorbium 200.
- **Excruciating pain in open cancer such as cancer of mouth, lips.** Calcarea Acetica 200.
- **In lung cancer and if there is sharp pain which radiates from the chest into the back. Chest very sensitive to touch.** Calcarea Carb 200.
- **Pain and foul smell or stench coming from the affected area.** Cinnamonum mother tincture. Give 10 drops every hour.
- **Pain in case of stomach cancer.** Give Condurango mother tincture, 10 drops every hour.
- **Piercing pain in tumours, worse at night.** Conium 1000.
- **Pain in cancerous tumours and ulcers.** Hydrastis 200.

- **Pain causes twitching or jerking of limbs. Patient cannot bear the pain.** Morphinum 200.

You may give more than one medicine. The aim is to reduce the suffering of the patient to the extent possible.

**Conclusion**

**Cancer, particularly in advanced stages is almost incurable. We have to accept that fact. All we can do is to try to reduce the suffering of the patients and enable them to live as normal a life as possible.** The dosage of medicine given here are indicative. Feel free to increase dosage if it relieves the suffering of the patient.

# Epilogue

**Grandpa says that all persons must strive to be healthy. Just as there are many roads to Rome, there are many ways of staying healthy. Some may go to the gym. Others may opt for Yoga. Some may believe in being veggie. Others may go for high protein non-vegetarian diet. But to be healthy, all must eat healthy, opt for a healthy life style and learn to cope with stress. The focus should be on prevention and early detection of diseases and treatment. Grandpa shares his knowledge and experience in this book.**

**Grandpa has used Homeopathy for the last 35 years to prevent and treat medical problems.** Homeopathy provides us a life line in emergencies and serious illnesses till we can reach competent medical aid i.e., a doctor or a hospital as the case may be. **Limitations of Homeopathy have been clearly explained in Chapter 2 of this book. Serious problems must be referred to a doctor.**

In case of suspected serious illness or injury, it is best to see an allopathic doctor of repute. This is because the allopathic doctors rely more on medical investigations like X-Ray, biopsy tests, blood tests, etc for their diagnosis. Hence their diagnosis is likely to more accurate than one which is done without tests. **Do not go to a Homeopathic, Unani or Ayurveda doctor in case of life-threatening diseases like heart attacks, problems of the kidney or liver, appendicitis, typhoid, tuberculosis, dengue, chikungunya, malaria etc.** Practitioners of traditional or Homeopathic medicine may delay proper investigation and try to treat the problem without a proper investigation. This may result in the treatment getting fatally delayed.

After you have seen a doctor of your choice and done any investigations that he had recommended, the doctor will come up with a diagnosis and a recommended a line of treatment. He will prescribe medicines or recommend hospital admission. The patient should study the medical problem as diagnosed on the internet. The patient and his family will then have a clear picture about the seriousness of the disease, the expenses involved and the logistic problems and decide what to do keeping in mind the age of the patients and the financial status of the family. **Grandpa does not believe that it is correct to reduce the young to living dead by spending more than one can afford in trying to save the life of an aged or terminally ill person. An article in Times of India published recently stated that about**

**ten million Indians are reduced to poverty every year because of money spent on medical expenses. The willingness to accept death as a part of life and reliance on Homeopathy can substantially reduce that number.**

Homeopathic self-medication or treatment is reasonably safe and simple. It is cheap and free from side effects. It also provides options to ladies and others who feel shy to discuss their intimate sexual or psychological problems. It can provide a life-saving solution if you cannot afford expensive medical treatment. **All those who travel, live or work in areas where medical aid is not easily available would be advised to buy this book (down load on to lap tops), study this book carefully and keep a medical kit as suggested in Chapter 2.**

To obtain maximum benefit from the book you should:

- Study Chapters 1 to 5 and get an understanding eating healthy and of Homeopathy and glance through the rest of the book and make yourself familiar with it.
- **Note medicines which are inimical to each other.** Refer to it if you are using more than one medicine at the same time.
- Acquire the medicine kit unless you live in a town where Homeopathic medicines are easily available.
- Use the content and index at the end of the book to find the appropriate medicine or medicines that address your problem and start the course.
- **If there is no improvement within three days, the medicine selected is not appropriate or the patient does not respond to Homeopathy. Try another medicine or go to a Homeopathy expert or seek a solution in a different stream of medicine.**

**In the end Grandpa would like to reiterate that this book is not a text book of Homeopathy. It is a manual for prevention, first aid and self-medication or in house medication till a patient can access expert medical treatment. It is also a manual for self-medication for minor or unusual problems which do not always require or respond to allopathic treatment. It is also a manual for self-medication for those who cannot afford allopathic treatment or where the doctor says that the patient is incurable.**

***All persons purchasing and using this book must realize that self-medication and Homeopathy has limitations which are explained in detail in Chapter 1. For all life- threatening diseases or injuries, the patient must be evacuated to a hospital at the earliest possible. The first aid or treatment***

***suggested is only a stop gap measure till expert medical facilities can be accessed. The author or the publisher does not accept any liability for self-medication or treatment suggested in the Boo***

## BIBLIOGRAPHY

1. Reader's Digest Medical Question and Answer Book
2. Lectures on Homeopathic Materia Medica by Dr. J. T. Kent
3. Materia Medica With Repertory by Dr. O. E. Boericke
4. Essentials of Homeopathic Therapeutics by Dr. W A Dewey
5. Homeopathic Guide to Family Health by R K Tandon and Dr. V. R. Bajaj
6. Beginners Guide to Homeopathy by T S Iyer
7. Clinical Relationship by Dr. Sukumar Roy
8. Dose and Potency by Dr. P S Rawat
9. www. homeocare.in
10. www. homeopathictreatment4u.com
11. www. homeopathyonline.in
12. www. abchomeopathy.com
13. www. holisticonline.com/homeopathy
14. www.drhomeo.com
15. www. e-homeopathy.com

## INDEX

A

Abortion: Ch. 16 Abscess: Ch. 15
Alcoholism: Ch. 18 Amnesia: Ch. 8 and 19
Anaemia: Ch. 16 Anal Problems: Ch. 13
Ankles: Ch. 7 and 14 Apathy: Ch. 8 and 19
Apoplexy: Ch. 7 and 8 Appendicitis: Ch. 11
Arthritis: Ch. 21 Asphyxiation: Ch. 7
Asthma: Ch. 7 and 10 Alzheimer Disease. Ch. 19

B

Back and Neck: Ch. 14 Barber's Itch: Ch. 15
Bad Breath: Ch. 9 Bashful: Ch 17
Bed Sores: Ch. 15 Bed Wetting: Ch. 20
Black Eye: Ch. 9 Bleeding: Ch 7
Blindness: Ch. 9 Blisters: Ch 15 and 18
Blood Pressure High: Ch. 10 Blood Pressure low: Ch 10
Boils/Carbuncles: Ch. 15 Breast Problems: Ch 16

Bruises: Ch. 15 Burns: Ch 7

C

Cancerous Substances: Ch 1 and 6 Cataract: Ch 1, 9 and 19
Cancer Stomach: Ch 22 Calves /Legs: Ch 14
Cancer Prostate: Ch 6 and 22 Cancer Throat: Ch 22
Cancer Blood/Leukaemia: Ch 22 Cancer Bone: Ch 22
Cancer Bowel: Ch 22 Cancer Breast: Ch 22
Cancer Cervix/ Ovary/Uterus: Ch 22 Cancer Food Pipe: Ch 22
Cancer Lungs: Ch 22 Cancer Mouth/Lips/Tongue: Ch 22
Cataract: Ch 1, 9, 19 Chicken Pox: Ch 20
Chills: Ch 8 Children's Diseases: Ch 20
Cholera: Ch 11 & 13 Cold/Coryza: Ch 10 & 20
Coma: Ch 7 & 8 Concussion: Ch 7
Conjunctivitis: p 51 Constipation: Ch 13 & 18
Corns/Callosities: Ch 14 Coronary Thrombosis Ch 10
Cough: Ch 10 & 20 Cracks in Skin: p 62
Cramps: Ch 13 & 19 Cuts/Punctured Wounds: Ch 7

D

Dangers of Self Medication: Ch 3 Debility: Ch 8
Dementia: Ch 8 & 19 Delirium: Ch 8
Depression: Ch 8 Detached Retina: Ch 9 & 19
Diabetes: Ch 11 Diabetic Gangrene: Ch 15
Digestive Systems: Ch 11 Diphtheria: Ch 10
Dosage of Medicines: Ch 3 Dog Bite: Ch 7
Dysentery: Ch 13 Dyspepsia: Ch 18

E

Eating Healthy: Chapter 1 Eating for healthy eyes: Chapter 1
Ear Problems: Ch 9 Eczema: Ch 15
Encephalitis: Ch 8 Epilepsy: Ch 8
Eructation: Ch 11 Erysipelas: Ch 15
Exposure: Ch 8 Eye Problems: Ch 1, 9 & 19

F

Face: Ch 8 Fear: Ch 8
Fatty Liver Disease: Ch 18
Feet: Ch 14 Fevers: Ch 8
First Aid: Ch 7 First Aid for Apoplexy or Stroke: 7
First Aid for Appendicitis: Ch 7 First Aid for Asphyxiation: Ch 7
First Aid for Asthma Attack: Ch 7 First Aid for Black Eye: Ch 7

First Aid for Burns and Scalds: Ch 7 First Aid for Coma: Ch 7
First Aid for Cramps: Ch 7 First Aid for Cuts or Wounds: Ch 7
First Aid for Dog Bite: Ch 7 First Aid for Ear Ache: Ch 7
First Aid for Encephalitis: Ch 7 First Aid for Epileptic Fits: Ch 7
First Aid for External Bleeding: Ch 7 First Aid for Food Poisoning: Ch 7
First Aid for Foreign Bodies: Ch 7 First Aid for Fracture: Ch 7
First Aid for Frostbite: Ch 7 First Aid for Heart Attack: Ch 7
First Aid for Heat Stroke: Ch 7 First Aid for Injury to Back: Ch 7
First Aid for Injury to Eye: Ch 7 First Aid for Injury to Nerves: Ch 7
First Aid for Insect Bites: Ch 7 First Aid for Internal Bleeding: Ch 7
First Aid for Pains: Ch 7 First Aid for Shock: Ch 7
First Aid for Snake Bite: Ch 7 First Aid for Sprains and Strains: Ch 7
First Aid for Toothache: Ch 7 Flatulence/Gas: Ch 11
Food Poisoning: Ch 11 Foreign Bodies: Ch 7
Frostbite: Ch 7 & 15 Fundamentals of Homeopathy Ch 2

G

Gall Stones: Ch 11 Gangrene: Ch 15
Glaucoma: Ch 9 &b19 Gout: Ch 21

H

Hair Problems: Ch 8 Hand Problems: Ch 14 & 18
Hallucination: Ch 8 Hangover: Ch 18
Headache: Ch 8 Hearing Loss: Ch 9 & 19
Heart Problems: Ch 6, 7 & 10 Heart Attack: Ch 6, 7 & 10
Heat Stroke: Ch 7 Heel problems: Ch 14
Herpes: Ch 15 Hip Problems: Ch 14
Homeopathic Kit: Ch 4 Homeopathic Medicines: Ch 4
Hysteria: Ch 8 Hydrocele: Ch 17

I

Impotence: Ch 17 Incompatibility of Medicines: Ch 4 Influenza/Flu: Ch 6 & 8 Injury: Ch 7
Insect Bites and Stings: Ch 6 & 15 Insomnia: Ch 6, Ch 18
Intermittent Fevers: Ch 8 Irritable: Ch 8 & 19
Itching: Ch 15

J

Jaundice: Ch 6 & 11

K

Kidney Stones: Ch 6 & 12 Knees: Ch 14 & 21

L

Lack of Determination: Ch 8 Laryngitis: Ch 9
Leg Problems: Ch 14 Leukoderma: Ch 15
Leucorrhoea: Ch 16 Leukaemia: Ch 22
Lice: Ch 8 Lip Problems: Ch 9
Liver Problems: Ch 11 & 18 Loss of Hearing: Ch 9 & 19
Lung Problems: Ch 10 Life Style Problems Ch 18

M

Mania: Ch 8 Measles: Ch 6 & 8
Melancholy: Ch 8 & 19 Memory Loss: Ch 8 & 19
Meningitis: Ch 8 Menopause: Ch 16
Menstruation Problems: Ch 16 Migraine: Ch 18
Motion Sickness: Ch 8 Morning Sickness: Ch 16
Mouth Problems: Ch 9 Mumps: Ch 6 and 8
Myths and Realities: Ch 5 Myasthenia Gravis: Ch 14

N

Nails: Ch 14 Neck Problems: Ch 14 & 18
Nightmares: Ch 8 Nipples: Ch 16
Noise in Ears: Ch 9 Nose Problems: Ch 9
Numbness: Ch 14 Nymphomania: Ch 17

O

Obesity: Ch 18 Odour: Ch 15
Old Age Problems: Ch 1 & 19 Ovary Problems: Ch 16

P

Pain Chest: Ch 7 & 10 Pain Elbow: Ch 14 & 18
Pain Stomach: Ch 11 Pain Tail Bone: Ch 14 & 18
Pain Teeth: Ch 9 Pain Urinating: Ch 12
Palpitation: Ch 10 Paralysis Extremities: Ch 14
Paralysis Face: Ch 8 Parkinson's Disease: Ch 19
Perspiration: Ch 15 Pharyngitis: Ch 9
Phimosis; Ch 20 Piles: Ch 13 & 18
Pimples: Ch 8 & 15 Pneumonia: Ch 10
Polio: Ch 6 Polyps: Ch 15 & 16
Pregnancy Problems: Ch 16 Premature Ejaculation: Ch 17
Prevention of Abortion: Ch 6 & 16 Prevention of Bad Breath: Ch 6 & 9
Prevention of Cholera: Ch 6 Prevention of Colds: Ch 6
Prevention of Diarrhoea: Ch 6 Prevention of Diphtheria: Ch 6
Prevention of Erysipelas: Ch 6 Prevention of Fear: Ch 6 & 8
Prevention of Hangover: Ch 18 Prevention of Hay Fever: Ch 6

Prevention of Heart Problems: Ch 1 & 6 Prevention of Influenza: Ch 6
Prevention of Insomnia: Ch 6 Prevention of Intermittent Fevers: Ch 6 &
8
Prevention of Measles: Ch 6 Prevention of Motion Sickness: Ch 16
Prevention of Mumps: Ch 6 Prevention of Pus Formation: Ch 7
Prevention of Suicide: Ch 6 & 8 Prevention of Sweating: Ch 15
Prevention of Tetanus: Ch 6 Prevention of Tonsillitis: Ch 6 & 9
Prevention of Whooping Cough: Ch 6 Prickly Heat: Ch 15
Pain Back: Ch 14 Prostrate Problems: Ch 1, 6, 12 & 19
Psychological Problems: Ch 8 & 16

R

Rheumatism: Ch 21 Ring Worms: Ch 15
Running Nose: Ch 9 Retina Problems: Ch 1, 9 & 19

S

Sciatica: Ch 14 Selection of Medicines: Ch 4
Shock: Ch 7 and 8 Shoulders: Ch 14
Sinusitis: Ch 9 Skin Problems: Ch 15
Sleep Problems: Ch 6 & 8 Sneezing: Ch 9
Snoring: Ch 9 Spondylosis: Ch 14
Sprains: Ch 7 & 14 Spurting Stool: Ch 13
Squint: Ch 9 Stagger: Ch 14
Stammer: Ch 9 Stomach Pain: Ch 11
Stomach Upset: Ch 11 & 13 Stool Problems: Ch 13
Strains: Ch 14 Stroke: Ch 7 and 8
Stress Management: Ch 1 & 18 Sexual Problems Ch 17
Stys: Ch 9 Sweating: Ch 15

T

Typhoid: Ch 8 Teeth and Gums: Ch 8
Testicles Retracted: Ch 17 Tetanus: Ch 6
Thighs Problems: Ch 14 Thrombosis: Ch 6 & 10
Throat Problems: Ch 9 Toe Problems: Ch 14
Tongue: Ch 9 Tonsillitis: Ch 9 & 20
Tuberculosis: Ch 8 and 10 Tumour: Ch 11 & 16
Twitching and Trembling: Ch 14 & 19

U

Ulcer: Ch 11 and 16 Under Developed Breasts: p 67
Urinary Problems: Ch 12 Uterus Problems: Ch 16
V

Varicose Veins: Ch 16 and 19 Vertigo: Ch 8
Vomiting: Ch 11

W

Warts: Ch 15 Women's problems: Ch 16
Whitlow: Ch 14 Whooping Cough: Ch 6 and 20
Worms: Ch 20 Wrist and Arm: Ch 14

## *About the Author*

Col (Retd) Bhaskar Sarkar VSM was born in 1940. He graduated in civil engineering from Kolkata University in 1963 and did post-graduation in Defence Studies at Defence Services Staff College, Wellington and in Management at College of Defence Management in Secundrabad 1983. He joined the Indian Army in 1963 and hung his boots after 28 years of distinguished service in the rank of Colonel. After retirement Col Sarkar joined the construction industry as a civil engineering and management consultant and served on many interesting projects. He was keen sportsman and his hobbies include wild life, gardening, travelling and charity work. A versatile writer, he has twelve published books in print and another 12"e" books and hundreds of articles. This is his fifth book in the "Grandpa Series"; the others being "Grandpa's Tips on Navigating Through Life"; "Grandpa's Tips on Management for All"; "Grandpa's Tales: Ambush and other Stories"; "Grandpa's Selection: Outstanding Victories of the Indian Army".

Other books by the Author are "Pakistan Seeks Revenge and God Saves India"; "Tackling Insurgency and Terrorism"; "Kargil War, Past Present and Future": "Thirty-nine Steps to Happiness": "Practical Approach to Vaastu Shastra"; "Earthquakes"; "Nationalism: Economic Strategy for Survival of Developing Countries"; "An Introduction to Religions of the World"; "Who is Afraid of the Chinese Dragon? I am"; "Tackling the Maoist Menace". Bhaskar Sarkar's Author Profile on Smashwords is: www.smashwords.com/profile/view/Bhaskarsarkar1940 .

9 798887 832845

Printed by Libri Plureos GmbH in Hamburg,
Germany